STILL A BIT WONKY

A record of the lived experience of Dementia

Pat Simmons

Published by the Power Writers Publishing Group in 2025.

ISBN: 978-1-7638925-8-3 Print

ISBN: 978-1-764276 1-0-8 eBook

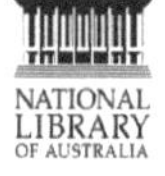

A catalogue record for this work is available from the National Library of Australia

Cover by Andrew Davies.

Internal layout by Joel Annesley.

Edited by Jane Turner.

Introduction

The image on the cover of this book is that of our father, Jack Irving Edwardes, who was born on October 21st, 1923. His parents, Colman Irving Edwardes and Florence Edwardes, were music hall artists at The Palace Theatre in Birmingham at that time.

It's me next to Jack that you would have seen on the cover. I was three years old at the time.

I've written this book because I wanted to honour Jack in some way. He was a funny, kind, loving and generous husband, father, grandfather and friend to many people. I felt that sharing the artwork and the comments he recorded in his diaries over the seven years between being diagnosed with dementia and passing away would be a perfect way to do that.

I'm hoping the diary entries I've chosen, which represent Jack's way of handling his condition, might be of some comfort to others. Whether it's someone with a diagnosis of their own, or the loved ones and carers out there who have their own journey to manage, I feel that the legacy Jack has left should be available to anyone it could help.

Bringing this book into being has been a bittersweet experience for me. I went through the gamut of emotions as I was pulling this material together. There were times when I felt sad. There were also times when I felt proud, and others when I couldn't help smiling.

The only regret I have is that I didn't have the presence of mind to interview Jack when he was alive. It would have been a wonderful experience if we could have written his story together. He still had lots of long-term memories that would have made this book all the richer, and I would have learned more about his childhood, which I believe wasn't a happy one.

What I hope you get out of reading this book is a more optimistic take on dementia than you might have otherwise had. I say that because Jack was a happy and optimistic man who rather liked being told what to do, particularly by his wife, Babs. He relied on Babs for just about everything, including important instructions to write in his daily diary for the times when she was going out. These included household chores such as 'flip a duster', and basic things like 'sandwich in the fridge'. It's lovely to remember the way they communicated.

Thinking about my parents' relationship usually brings out that smile I mentioned earlier. There was never any doubt about the fact that Jack was totally devoted to Babs, just as she was devoted to him. That becomes clear in numerous diary entries.

A good example relates to a time when Babs had an accident and broke her wrist. Jack was beside himself with worry, possibly not only for Babs's well-being, but also for his own.

Jack was always the dreamer. Babs was also a dreamer, but she was a more practical one. For example, she was the person who ensured the finances were kept up to date. Meanwhile, Jack's constant dream of winning money is documented throughout his diary recordings. You'll see that his lotto/keno numbers are religiously noted.

This reminds me of the story I heard when I was very young. It was about Jack having bet the rent money on a horse. I imagine, much to everyone's relief, the horse won.

As I reflected on Jack's life every time I pulled his diaries out of the drawer, I hoped he knew just how much he was adored and respected. I also hope that when we teased him and affectionately called him 'wonky donkey', he knew that we loved him to bits. He had a wonderful sense of humour, and I'm grateful that a sense of humour is one of the gifts he bestowed on me, my sister Judy, and his grandchildren, Amy, Luke, Hannah and Samantha.

What I've done at the end of the book is include some images of Jack as a younger man, and some of the documents that will give you a sense of the man he was before he started writing in the diaries that have provided the majority of the material for this book.

The other thing I've done is use quotes from "Alice's Adventures in Wonderland" at the beginning of each chapter.

The quotes reflecting the changes Alice experienced during her mystical journey seem to match the changes Jack was experiencing during his dementia journey.

Among other things, I'm hoping that by sharing the lived experience of someone like Jack, I'll, in a sense, be giving dementia a face.

A MESSAGE TO DAD

Dear Dad,

More than once over the years, you said to me, 'We must sit down one day, and you can write my life story.'

'Yes, we must do that,' I'd say.

Sadly, we never got around to it. I wish we had, Dad. I'd know so much more about your early life.

But you have another story to tell now. The story you told over a seven-year period in your diaries.

I'm going to explain a few things to the readers as they make their way through this book, and I might add some comments here and there. But other than that, the stage is yours.

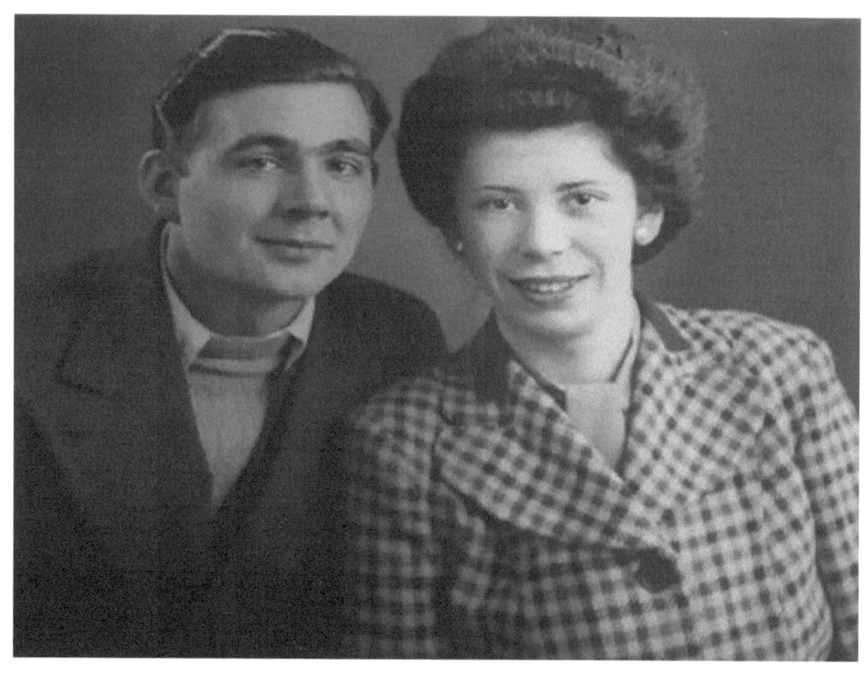

Mum and Dad

On February 4th, 1946, Jack married Barbara Hilda Tye – his beloved Babs, who supported him, loved him, and bought him a helluva lot of biros over the seven years of his dementia journey.

Chapter 1

2006

'What is the use of a book,' thought Alice, 'without pictures or conversation?'

June 20th

Jack's written down his lotto/keno numbers. He continued to do this for a number of years. For the record, no member of our family has ever won anything using these numbers, but good luck - dear reader!

Jack also regularly kept track of their bank balances.

I didn't know what S/W and L/W meant when I saw these letters in his diary, so I rang my sister Judy, to see if she knew, but she was as mystified as I was. What I did then was go through Jack's other diaries, and I found the answer — small wallet and large wallet.

The number 57 at the bottom of this first entry refers to the number of days Jack had been feeling 'wonky.'

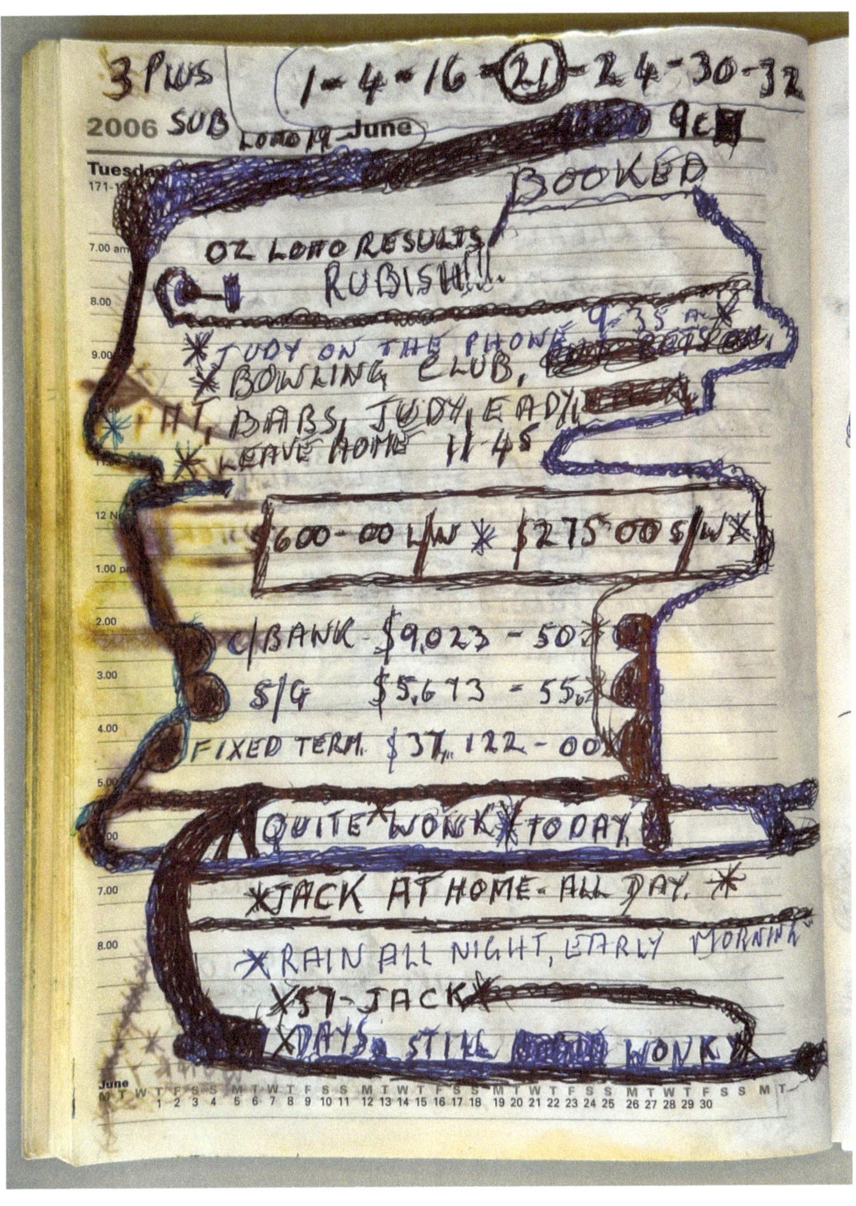
3 PLUS   1 - 4 - 16 - (21) - 24 - 30 - 32
2006 SUB   Lotto 19 June   9cm
Tuesday
171-
BOOKED
7.00 am
OZ LOTTO RESULTS
RUBISH!!!
8.00
9.00   * JUDY ON THE PHONE 9.35 A
BOWLING CLUB,
* PAT, BABS, JUDY, EADY
* LEAVE HOME 11.45
12 Noon
$600-00 L/W * $275.00 S/W
1.00 pm
2.00   C/BANK - $9,023 - 50
3.00   S/G $5,673 - 55
4.00   FIXED TERM $37,122 - 00
5.00
QUITE WONK * TODAY
* JACK AT HOME - ALL DAY. *
7.00
* RAIN ALL NIGHT, EARLY MORNING
8.00
X57-JACK
X DAYS, STILL WONK
June
M T W T F S S M T W T F S S M T W T F S S M T W T F S S M T W T F S S M T
1 2 3 4 5 6 7 8 9 10 11 12 13 14 15 16 17 18 19 20 21 22 23 24 25 26 27 28 29 30

August 17th

I can see from the original entry that Jack has blacked out some words by drawing over them. What's clear is that the lotto numbers were 'rubish'. These are words he writes a fair bit over the seven years his diaries cover.

He's counting the days since he started feeling 'wonky' and notes that Babs has gone shopping. I'm guessing she's asked Jack to do the washing up.

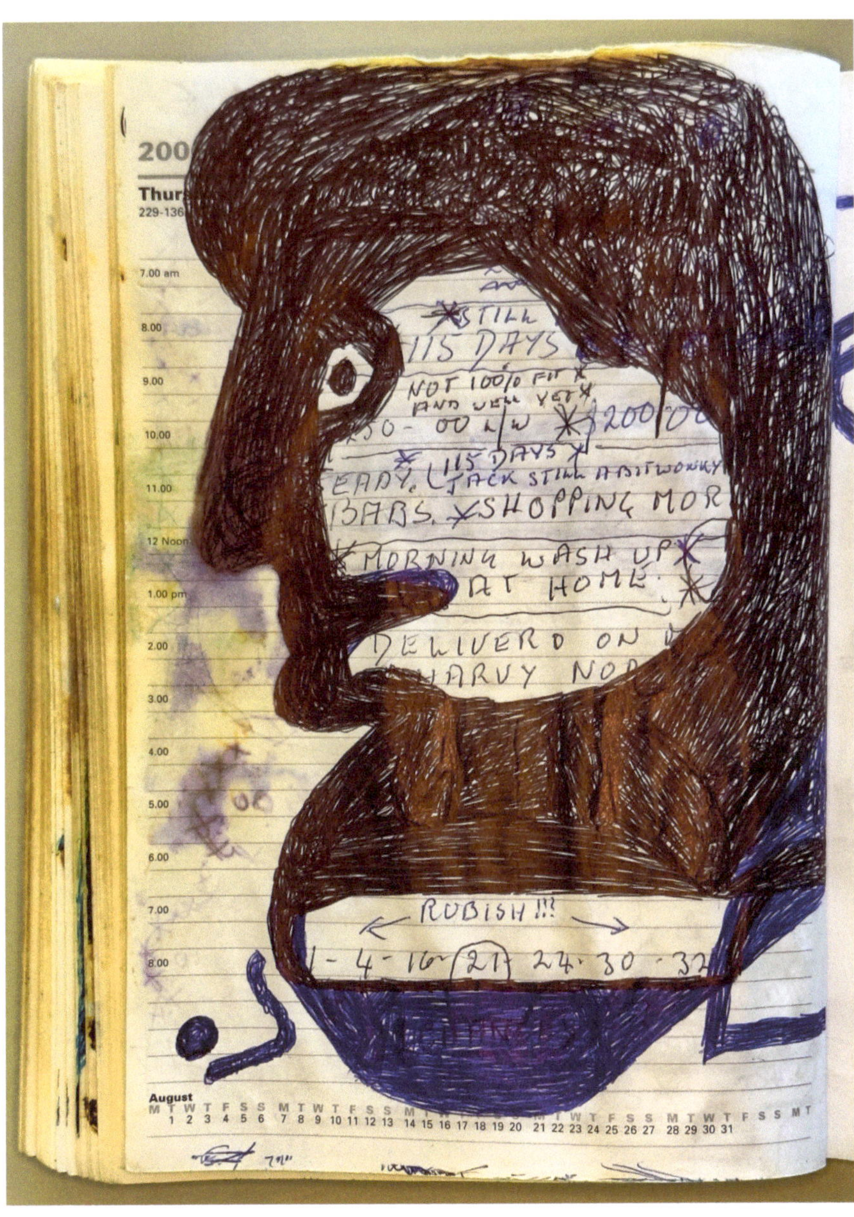
200
Thur
229-136
7.00 am
8.00
9.00
10.00
11.00
12 Noon
1.00 pm
2.00
3.00
4.00
5.00
6.00
7.00
8.00
STILL
115 DAYS
NOT 100% FIT
AND WELL YET
250 - 00 L/W $200 00
EADY. 115 DAYS
JACK STILL A BIT WONKY
BABS. SHOPPING MOR
MORNING WASH UP
AT HOME.
DELIVERD ON
HARVY NO
RUBISH !!!
1 - 4 - 16 21 24 30 32
August
M T W T F S S M T W T F S S M T W T F S S M T W T F S S M T
1 2 3 4 5 6 7 8 9 10 11 12 13 14 15 16 17 18 19 20 21 22 23 24 25 26 27 28 29 30 31

August 19th

'No bets on the horses today.'

I feel like Jack might have been struggling with how he was going to continue placing his bets.

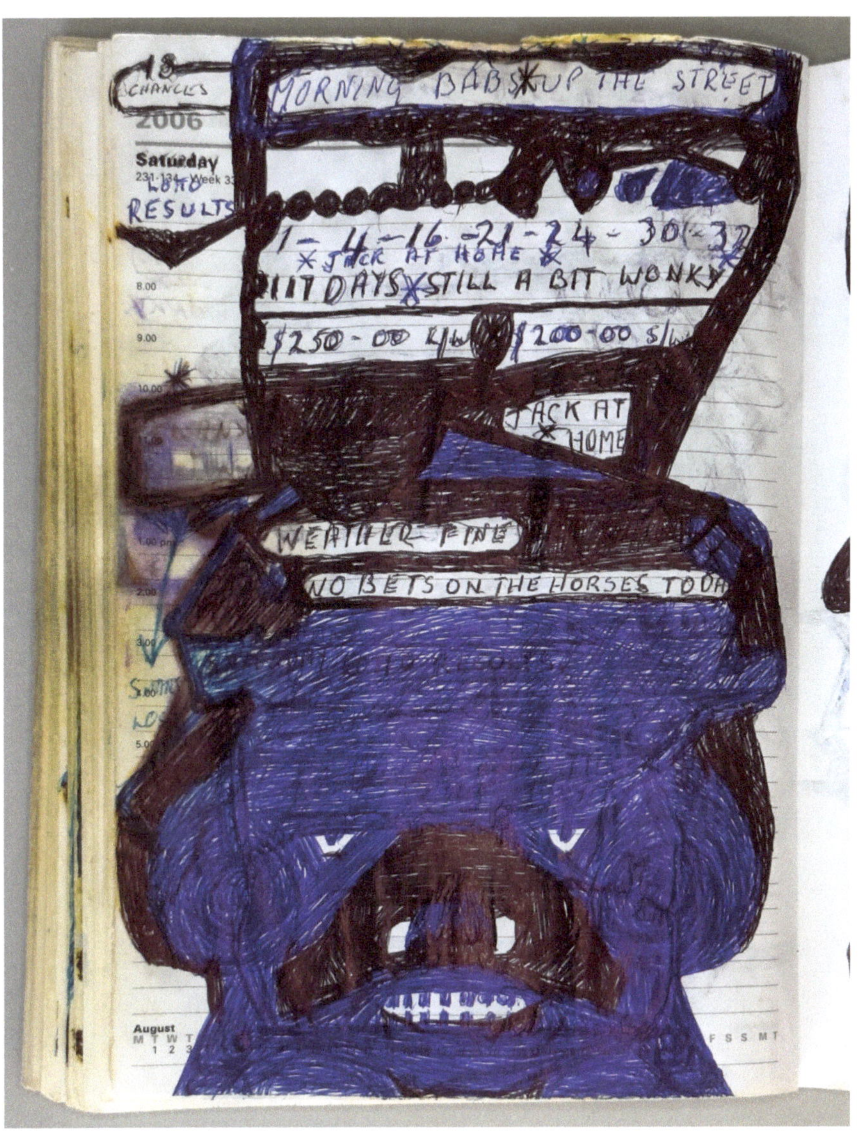
18
CHANCES
2006
Saturday
231-134 · Week 33
LONG
RESULTS
MORNING BABS * UP THE STREET
1 - 4 - 16 - 21 - 24 - 30 - 32
* JACK AT HOME *
BIT DAYS * STILL A BIT WONKY
$250 - 00 R/W * $200 - 00 S/W
JACK AT
* HOME
WEATHER FINE
NO BETS ON THE HORSES TODAY
August
M T W T   F S S M T
1 2 3

October 2nd

Jack mentions Eady at the bottom of the page. He always spells her name incorrectly. Edie was their next-door neighbour and a wonderful support for Babs. She and Babs would walk up to Engadine shops regularly to have a coffee and a chat.

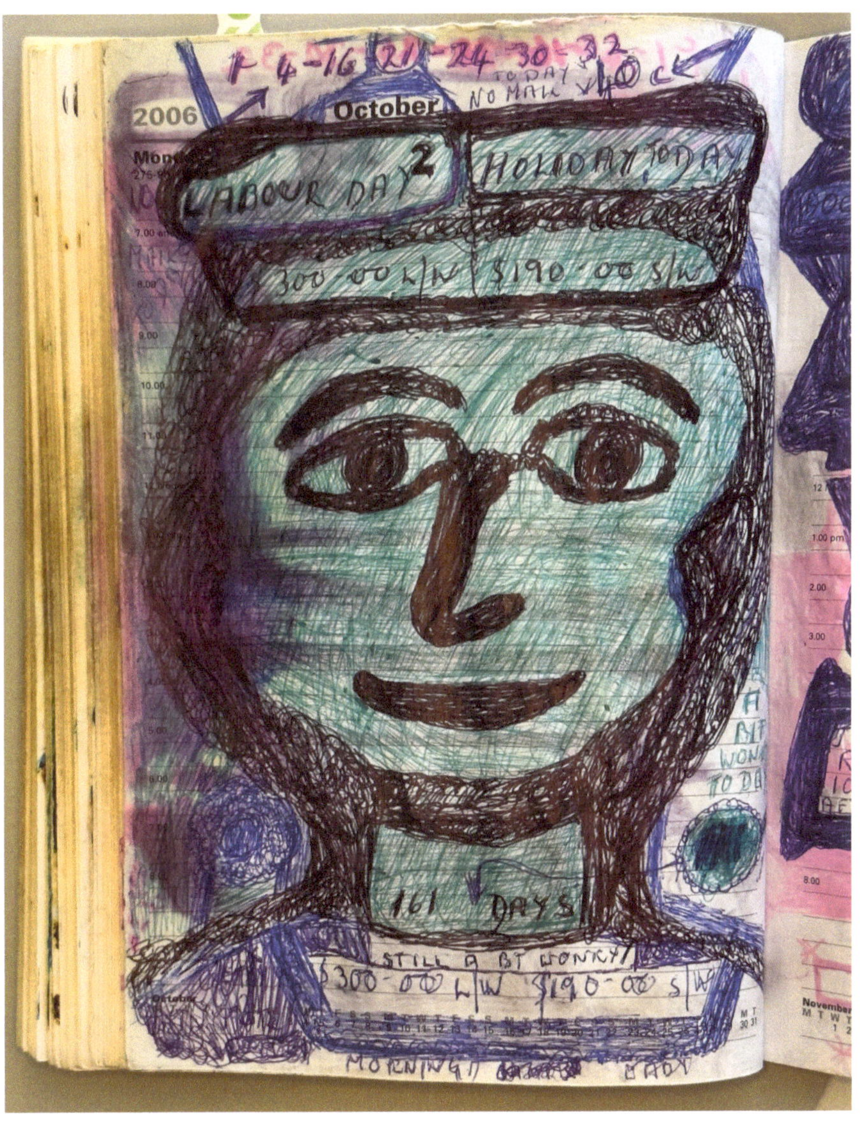
P 4-16 21-24 30-32
TODAY NO MAIL
2006 October
LABOUR DAY 2 HOLIDAY TODAY
300-00 L/W $190-00 S/W
161 DAYS
STILL A BT WONKY!
$300-00 L/W $190-00 S/W
MORNING!! LADY

October 7th

I love the fact that Jack has noted Babs had bought 'xmas puds' to put away. I find the image on the next page an interesting one. It's been suggested that it resembles a car crash by people I've shown it to. What do you think?

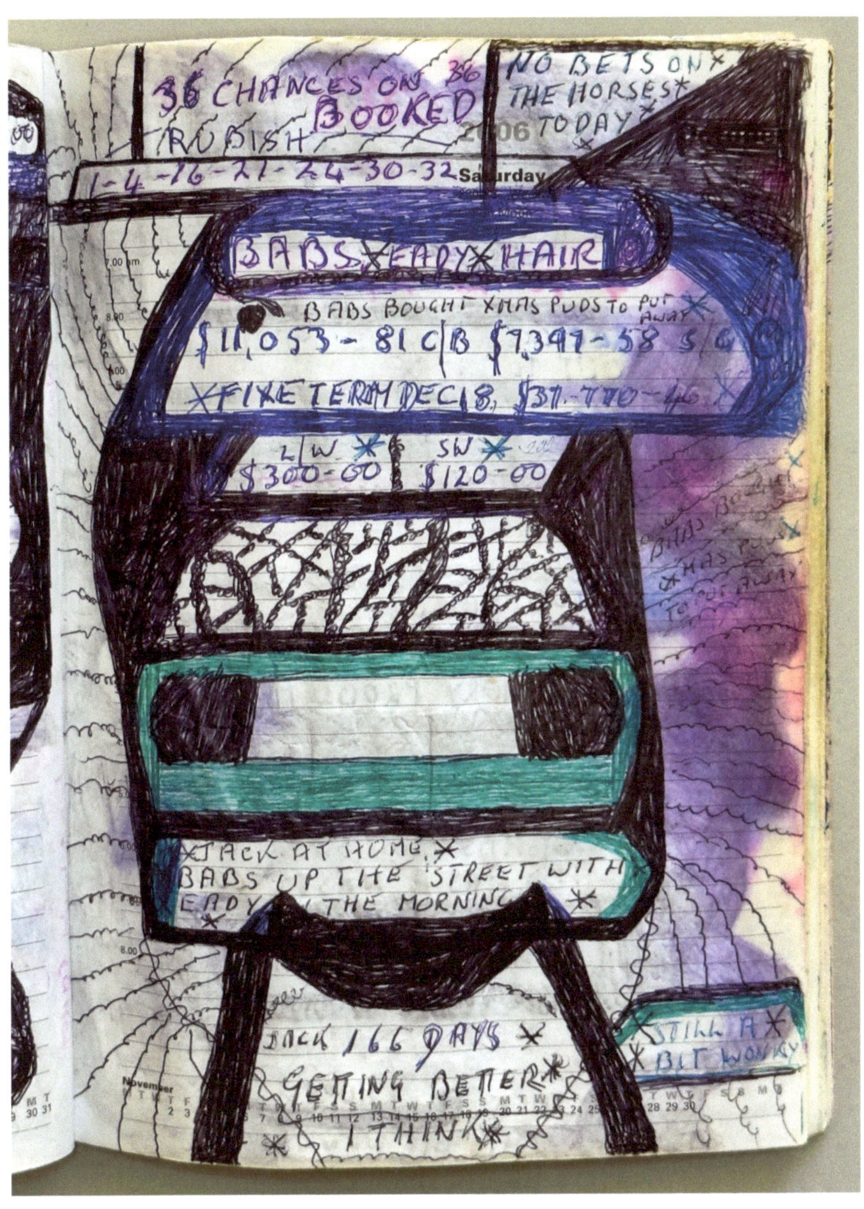
36 CHANCES ON 36
NO BETS ON
THE HORSES
BOOKED
TODAY
RUBISH
1 - 4 - 16 - 21 - 24 - 30 - 32
BABS EADY HAIR
BABS BOUGHT XMAS PUDS TO PUT AWAY
$11,053 - 81 C/B $7,397 - 58 S/C
FIXE TERM DEC 18, $31. 770 - 46
L/W $300 - 00   SW $120 - 00
JACK AT HOME.
BABS UP THE STREET WITH
EADY IN THE MORNING
JACK 166 DAYS
GETTING BETTER
I THINK
STILL A
BIT WONKY

November 27th

Jack and Babs lived in a small block of villas at Engadine, which is a suburb in the Sutherland Shire in Sydney. I note that Jeff, who is one of their neighbours, has taken Babs and Edie to Miranda (which is also in the Sutherland Shire) to shop.

I also note that Babs has left instructions for Jack to 'flip a duster' and do some housework, and let him know that there's a sandwich in the fridge for him to have for lunch.

It warms my heart to see that Jack recorded the fact that his granddaughter, Samantha, received 'the award of the year' at work.

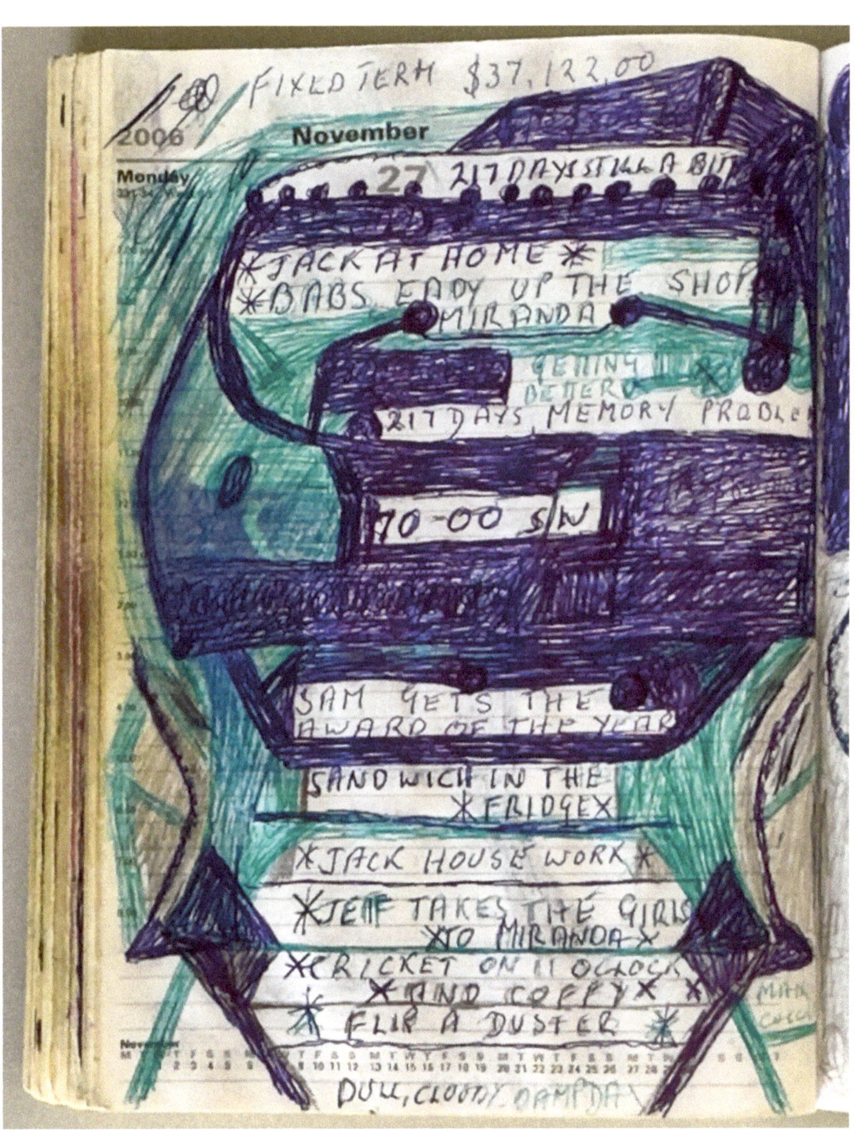
FIXED TERM $37,122,00
2006
November
Monday
27 217 DAYS STILL A BIT
JACK AT HOME
*BABS EADY UP THE SHOP
MIRANDA
GETTING
BETTER
217 DAYS MEMORY PROBLE
70-00 SW
SAM GETS THE
AWARD OF THE YEAR
SANDWICH IN THE
FRIDGE
JACK HOUSE WORK
*JEFF TAKES THE GIRLS
TO MIRANDA*
*CRICKET ON 11 OCLOCK
AND COFFY
FLIP A DUSTER
DULL, CLOUDY DAMP DAY

Chapter 2

2007

'Oh dear, how puzzling it all is! I'll try if I know all the things I used to know'

January 5th

Babs bought Jack lots of new pens for Christmas. I notice Jack has coloured over some of his writing. Who knows what that was about? There's no doubt that Jack gave his new pens quite a workout through the images you'll see over the next few pages though.

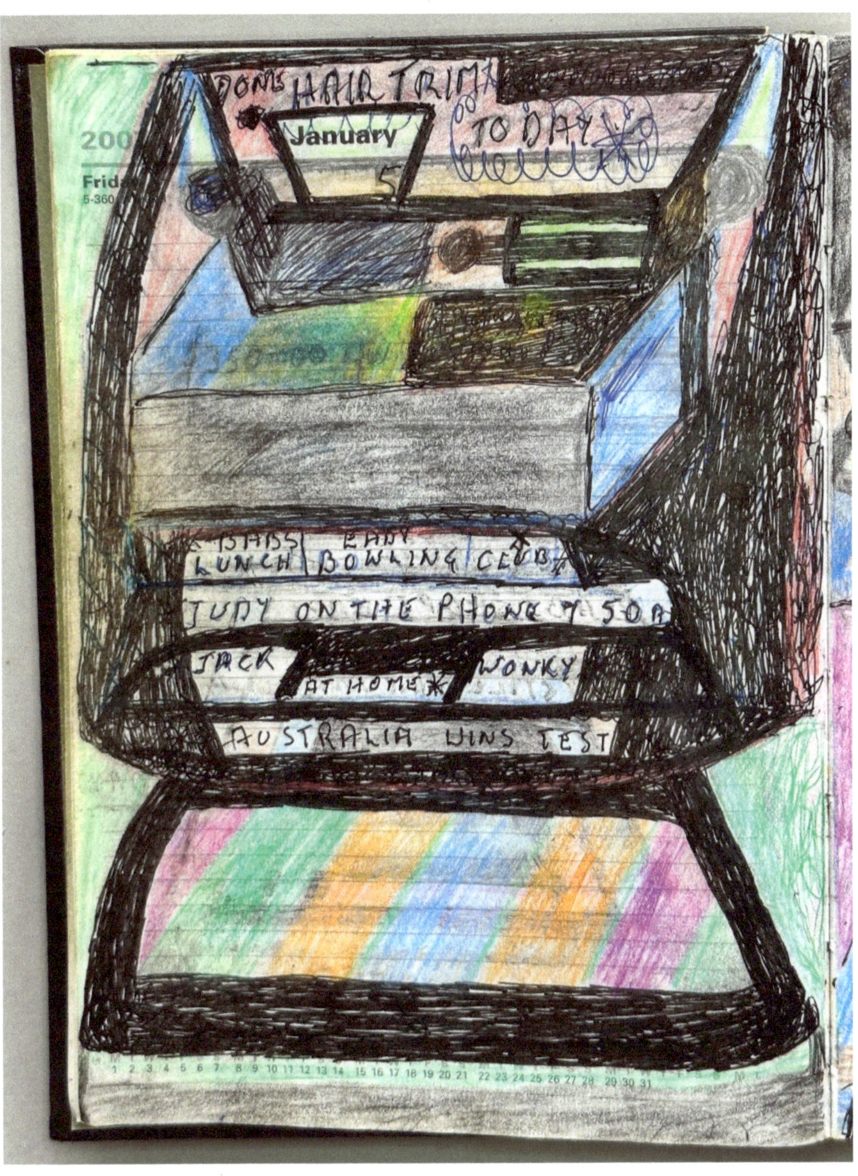
DONE HAIR TRIM
TODAY
200
January
5
Friday
5-360
BASS LUNCH EARLY
BOWLING CLUB
JUDY ON THE PHONE 7.50 A
JACK AT HOME WONKY
AUSTRALIA WINS TEST

January 27th

Jack's art has covered the date at the top of his diary page. As it was probably important for him to know the day and date each day, he's written 27 at the top of the page, and the day and date further down.

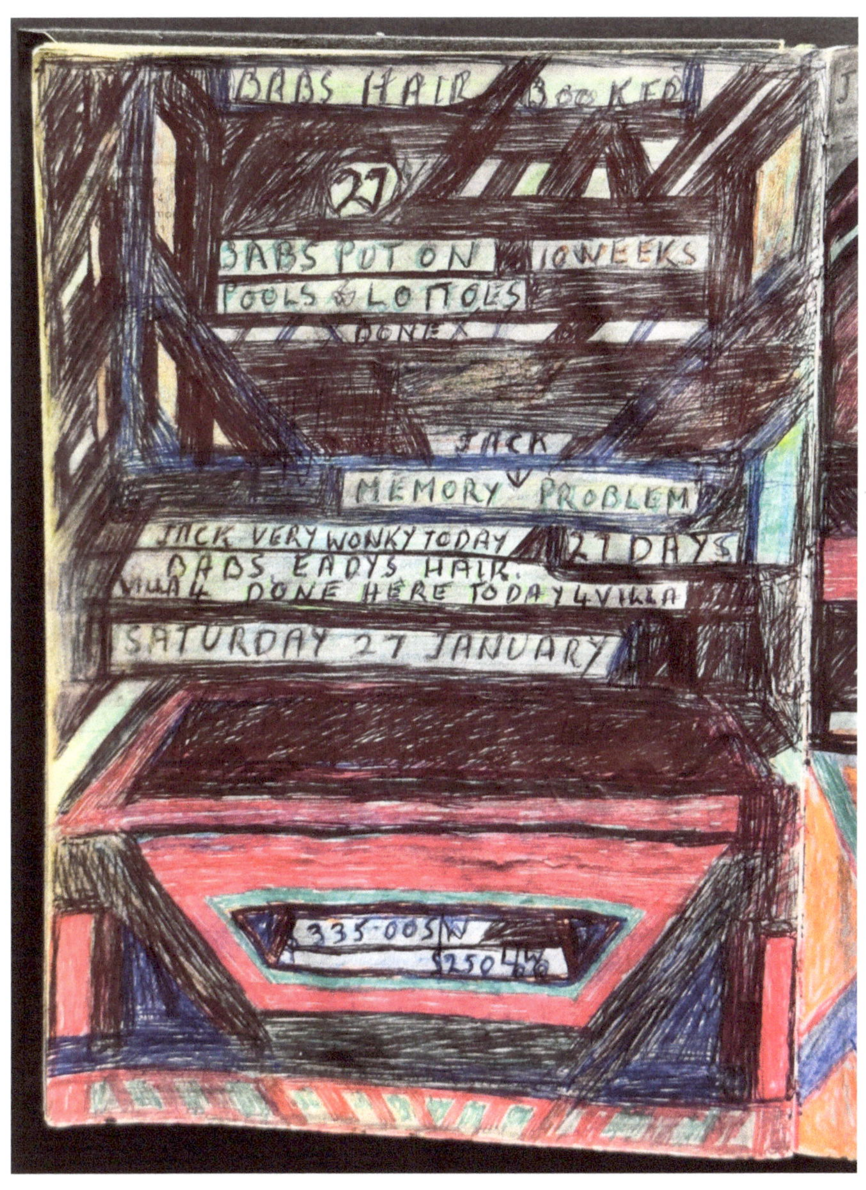
BABS HAIR BOOKED
27
BABS PUT ON 10 WEEKS
POOLS & LOTTOS
DONE
JACK
MEMORY PROBLEM
JACK VERY WONKY TODAY 27 DAYS
BABS EADYS HAIR.
VILLA 4 DONE HERE TODAY 4 VILLA
SATURDAY 27 JANUARY
335-0051 W
9250476

May 7th

There are a number of Jack's diary pages depicting windows – lots of windows. In the literary world, windows can represent things like a pathway to the outside world, freedom, and escape from limitations. At this point in time, Jack was still going out for walks with Babs, so he wasn't confined to remaining indoors, but I wonder whether, in his mind, he was starting to feel a sense of entrapment of some kind.

May
2 T DAYS MP
LOTTO RESULTS
$300-00 LW
$10 00 SW

May 17th

The main focus for Jack here was that the Lotto results are still 'RUBISH' – what's a typo among friends.

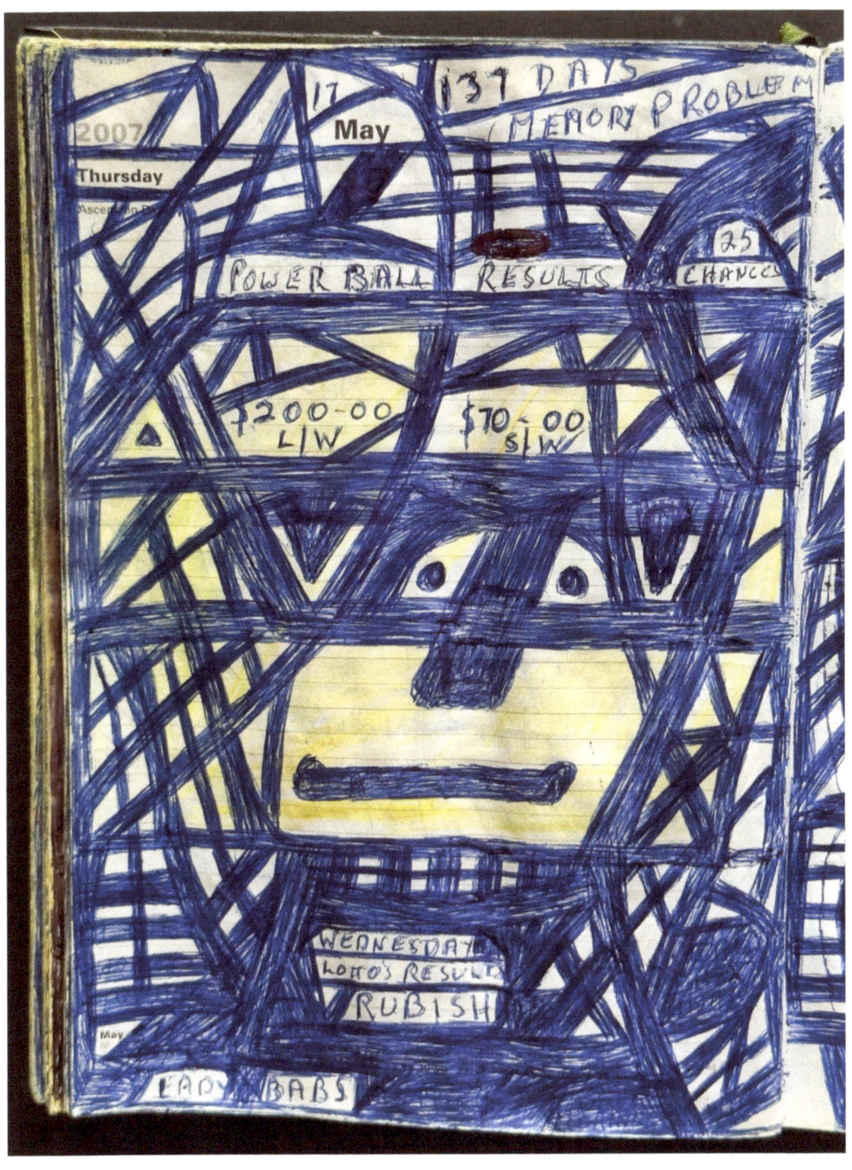
17
May
2007
Thursday
137 DAYS
MEMORY PROBLEM
POWER BALL RESULTS
25 CHANCES
$200-00 L/W
$70-00 S/W
WEDNESDAY
LOTTO'S RESULT
RUBISH
LADY BABS

June 4th

There aren't a lot of words here, but I feel like Jack might have had some fun colouring in the areas you'll see in the image opposite. Jack noted that if the weather was fine, he and Babs would have gone on a morning walk together.

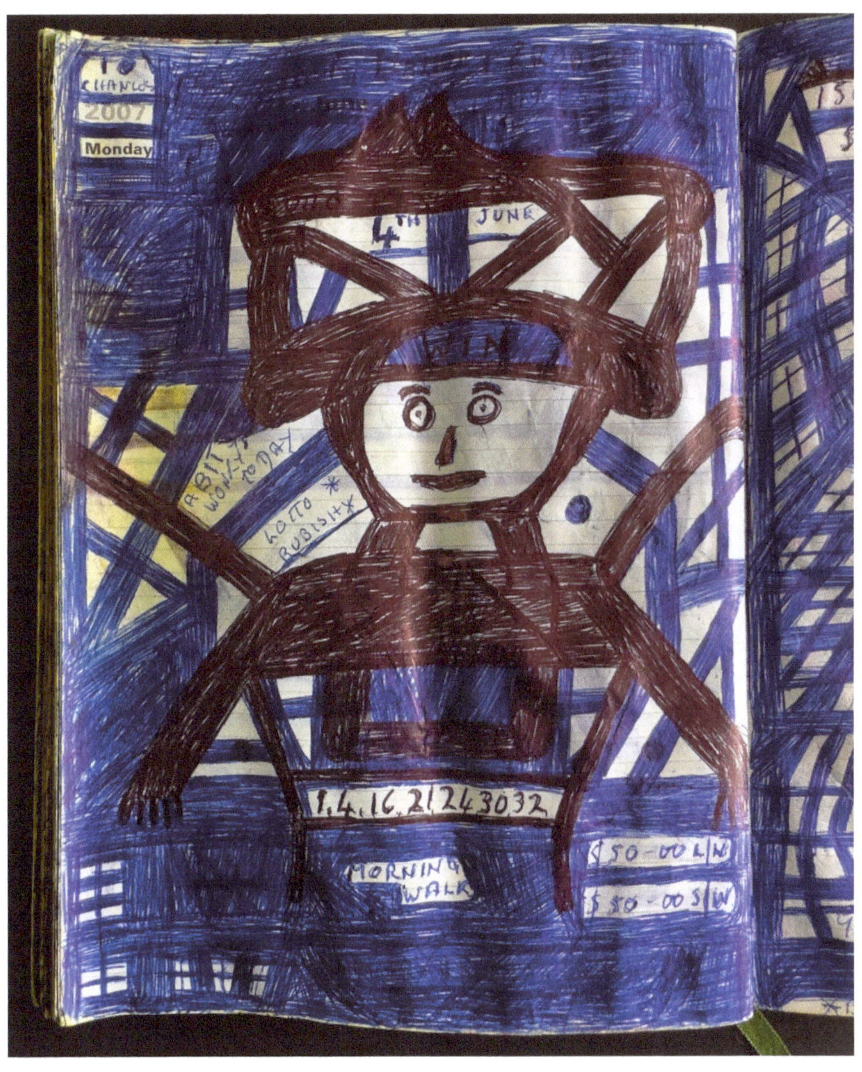
CHANCE
2007
Monday
4TH JUNE
A BIT
WON'T
TODAY
LOTTO
RUBISHY
1.4.16.21243032
MORNING WALK
$50-00 L/N
$50-00 S/W

August 22nd

I think Babs must have bought Jack some new red pens. You'll see more windows and some interesting triangles in the image on the next page. There are certainly a lot fewer words than you'll see on many of the other pages. I guess maybe Jack just didn't have a lot to say today.

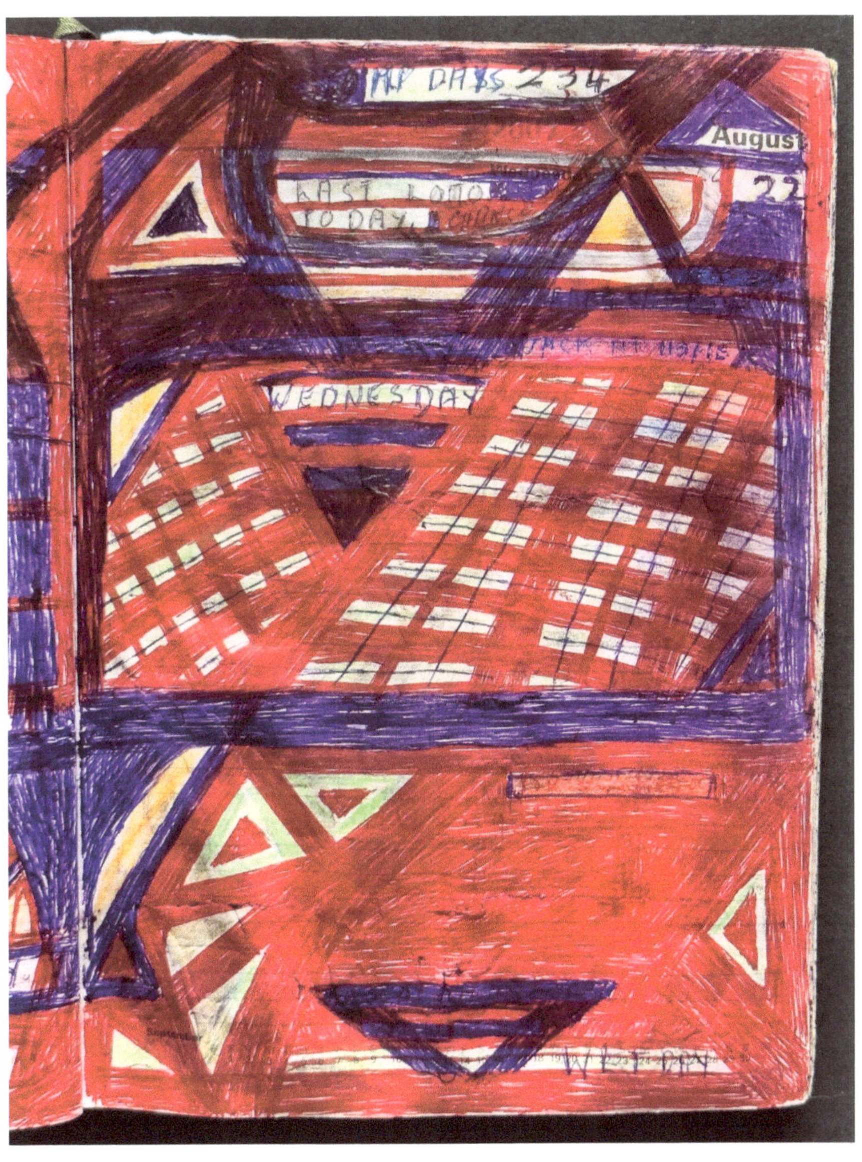
DAYS 234
August
22
LAST LONO
TO DAY
WEDNESDAY

September 3rd

Jack notes that he has 49 chances to win the Pools or Lotto – always the optimist. Many, many tiny windows are included on this page. Are they 'windows of opportunity'? Or do they represent the fact that a limited period of time exists when conditions make it possible for Jack to achieve a goal of some kind?

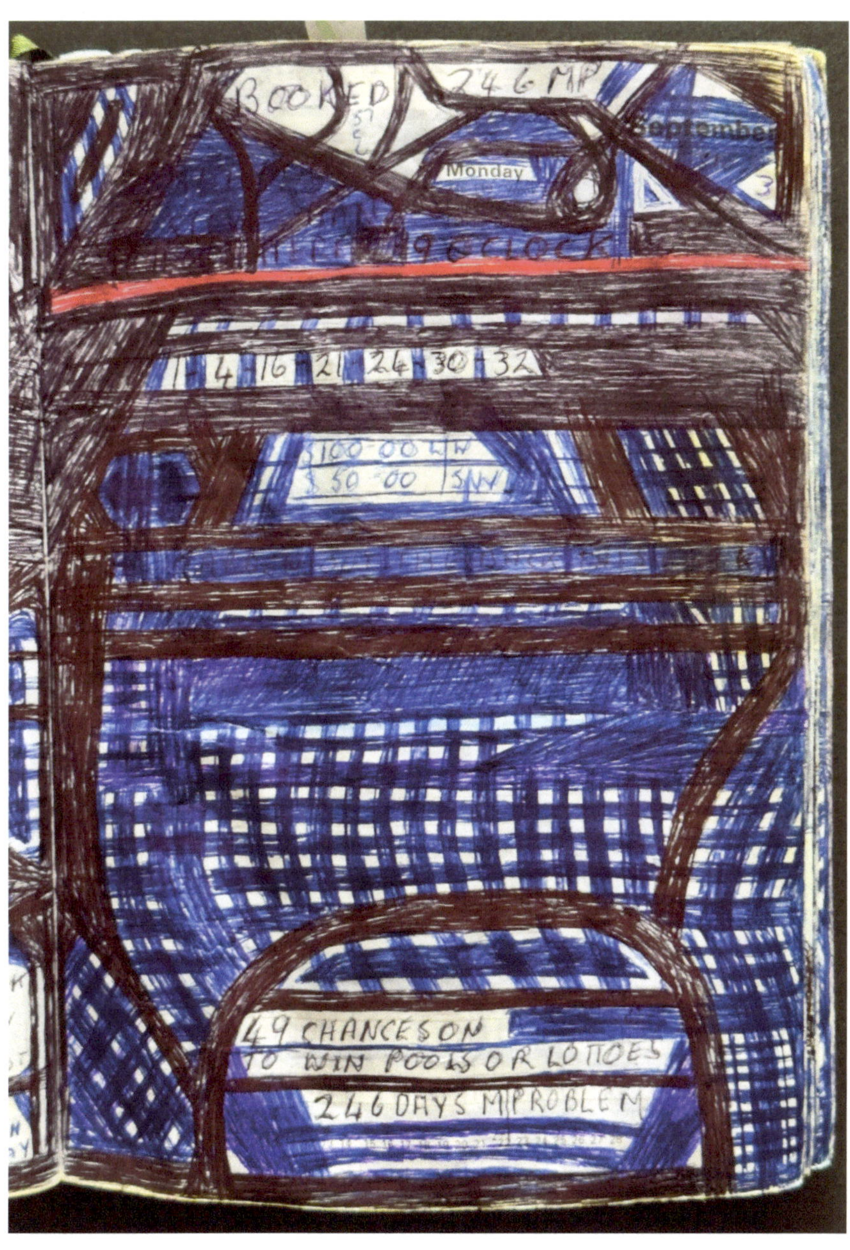

BOOKED 246 MP
September
Monday
3
9 OCLOCK
4 16 21 24 30 32
$100-00 WW
$50-00 SW
49 CHANCES ON
TO WIN POOLS OR LOTTOES
246 DAYS MY PROBLEM

September 16th

The entry on the opposite page has quite a different look to the images you've been seeing so far. It's both the colour and structure of the messages on this page that are notable from that point of view.

Again, the Lotto numbers are embedded in Jack's art. I don't know for sure, but I think he was drawing himself on this page.

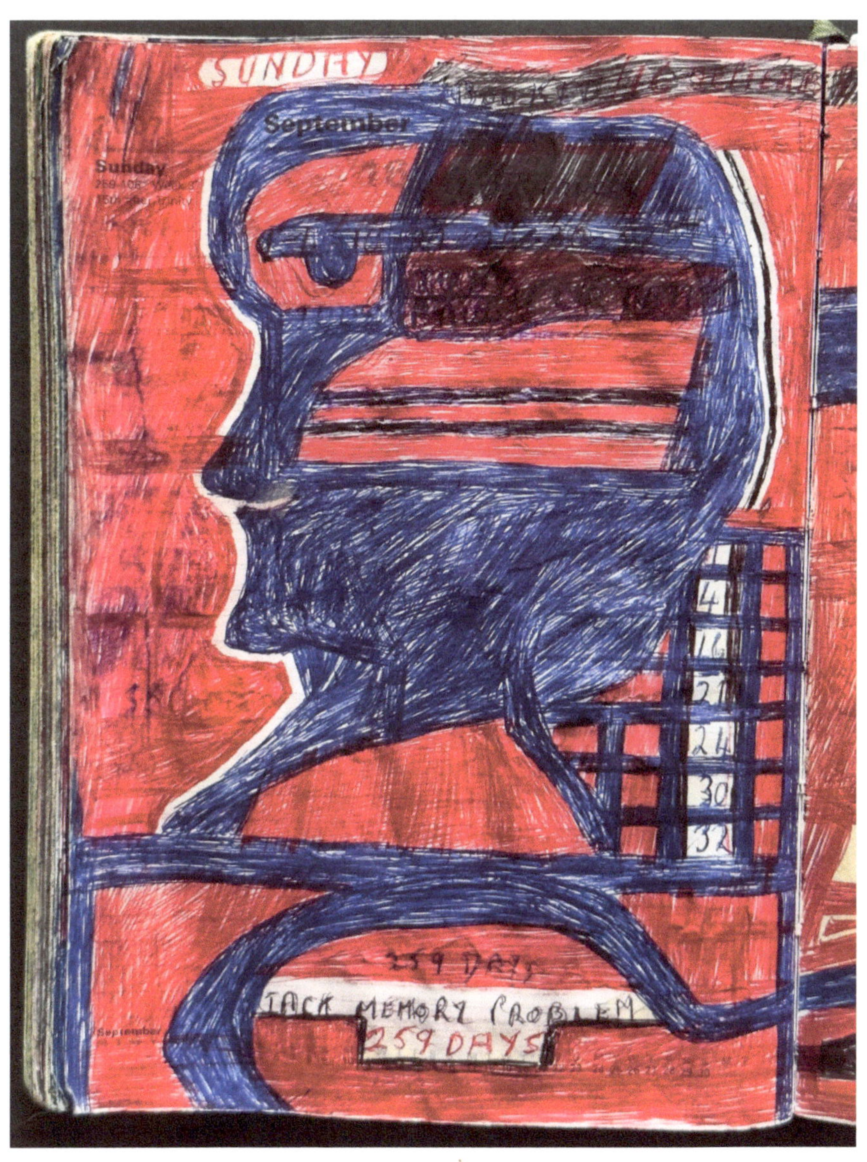
SUNDAY
September
Sunday
259 DAYS
JACK MEMORY PROBLEM
259 DAYS

Chapter 3

2008

'Curiouser and curiouser,' cried Alice

January 25th

This is a dark page in more ways than one. It's clear that Jack's struggling with the fact that Babs has broken her wrist, and he feels like more help is needed. That's probably because Jack never liked to see Babs unwell or hurt in any way.

It's interesting to note that some of the writing has been scribbled over. I wonder what it was that Jack didn't want to leave a record of by scribbling over the words.

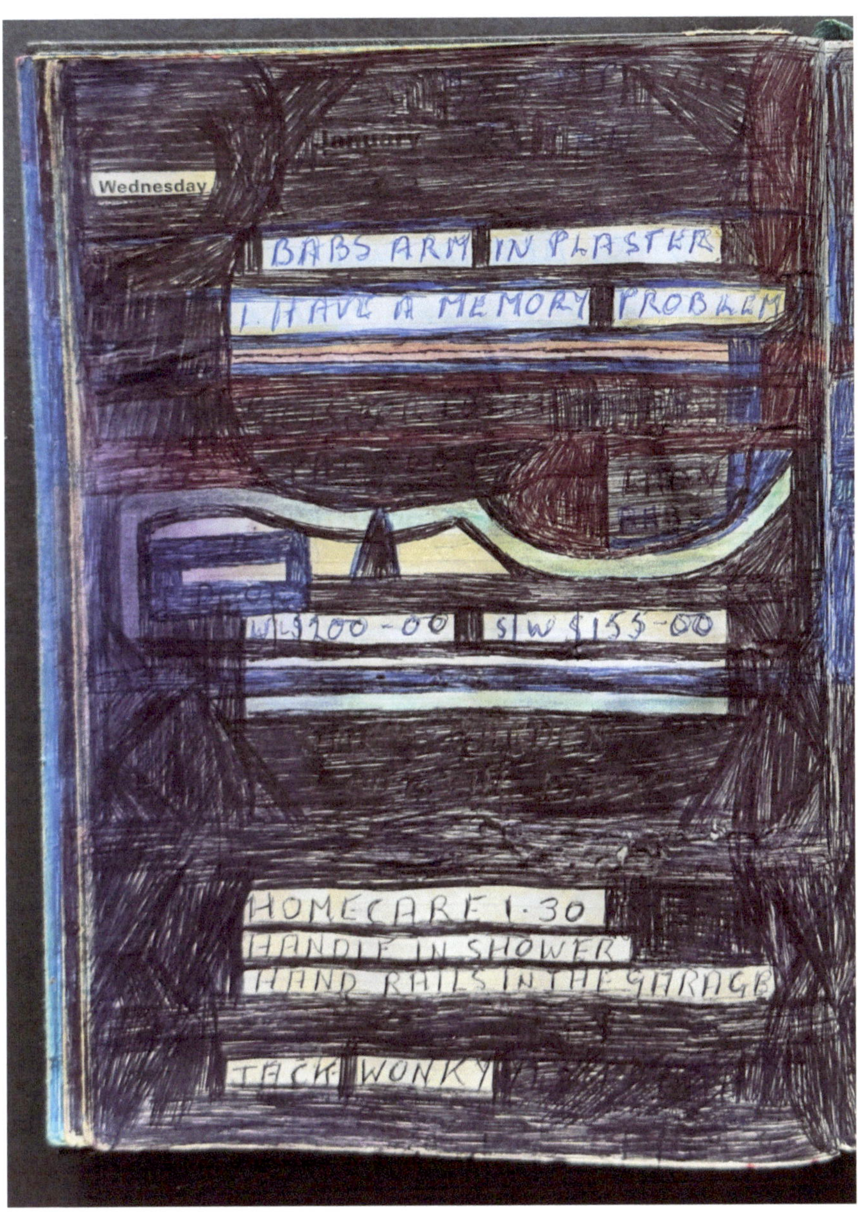
January
Wednesday
BABS ARM IN PLASTER
I HAVE A MEMORY PROBLEM
ML $200-00   S/W $155-00
HOMECARE 1.30
HANDLE IN SHOWER
HAND RAILS IN THE GARAGE
JACK WONKY

March 4th

Babs has managed to take some time out and have lunch at the Bowling Club today. You'll see that it's only black ink that is used on the next page, except for some light shading a third of the way down. I wonder if that reflected Jack's mood?

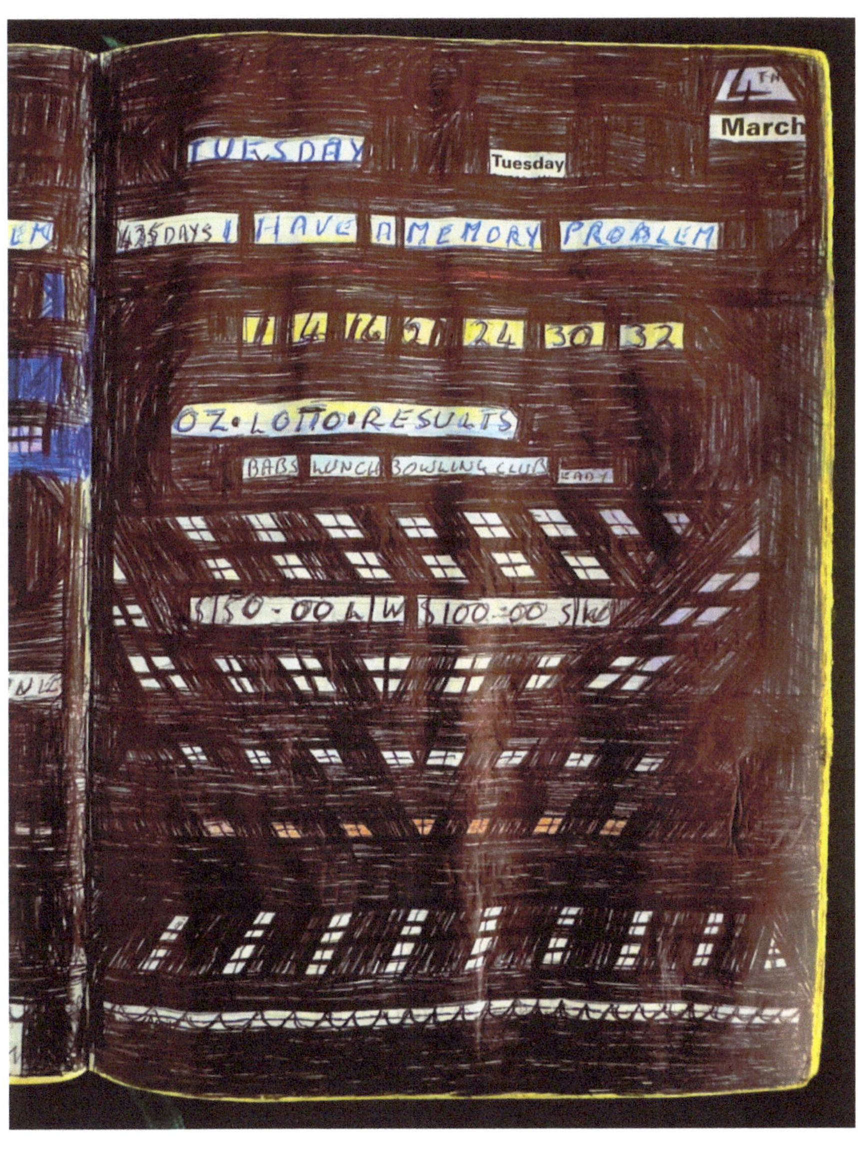
March
TUESDAY
Tuesday
435 DAYS I HAVE A MEMORY PROBLEM
11 14 176 6? 24 30 32
OZ·LOTTO·RESULTS
BABS LUNCH BOWLING CLUB LADY
$50·00 L/W $100·00 S/W

June 12th

Jack might be struggling with the fact that a hairdresser is going to be coming to the house to do Babs's hair today. As I've mentioned previously, he wasn't keen on having visitors unless they were friends or family.

I find it interesting that he's left a blank space on this page. I wonder what that means. I guess it's possible that he just ran out of things to say.

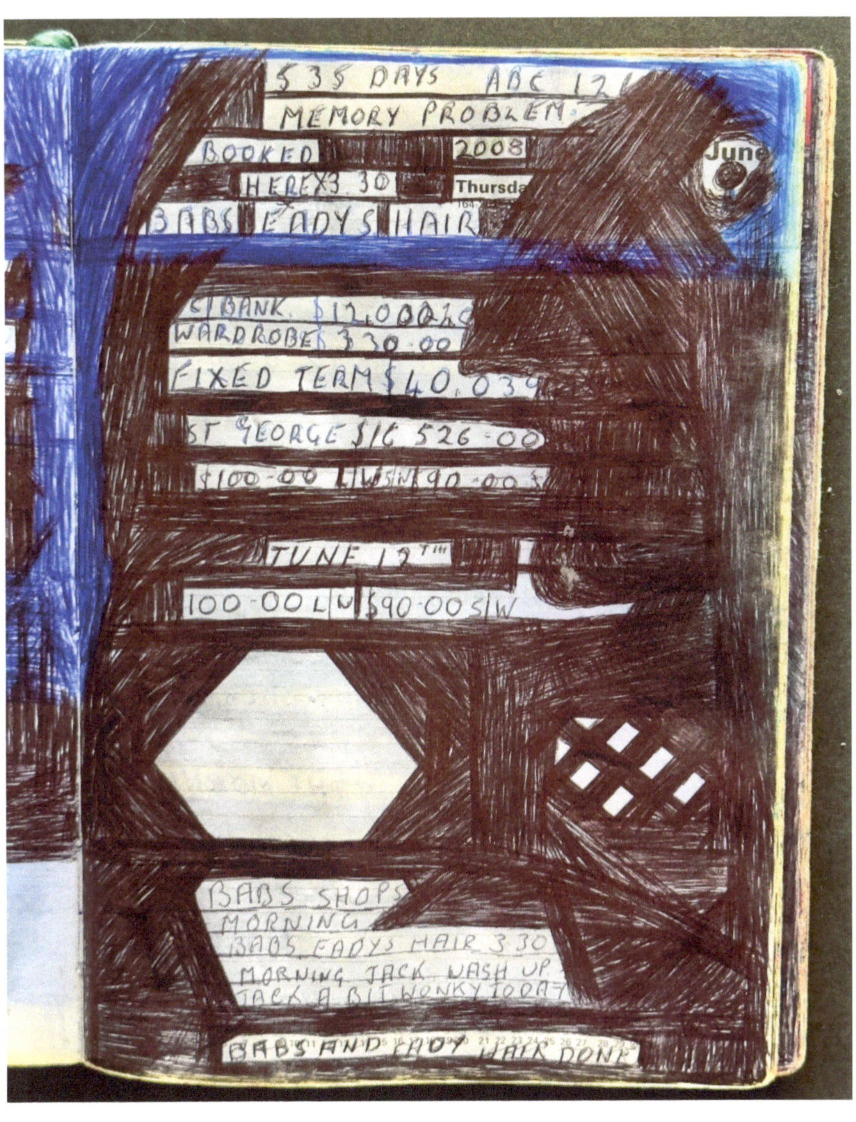
535 DAYS ABC 12
MEMORY PROBLEM
BOOKED 2008
HERE X3.30 Thursday
BABS EADYS HAIR
C/BANK $12,000.00
WARDROBE 330.00
FIXED TERM $40,039
ST GEORGE $16,526.00
$100.00 L/W $90.00 S/W
JUNE 12TH
100.00 L/W $90.00 S/W
BABS SHOPS
MORNING
BABS EADYS HAIR 3.30
MORNING JACK WASH UP
JACK A BIT WONKY TODAY
BABS AND EADY HAIR DONE

October 21st

It's Jack's 85th birthday today. Not only is there money in the small and large wallets, but there's also some in the wardrobe. It's lovely to see that he went out for lunch on his birthday.

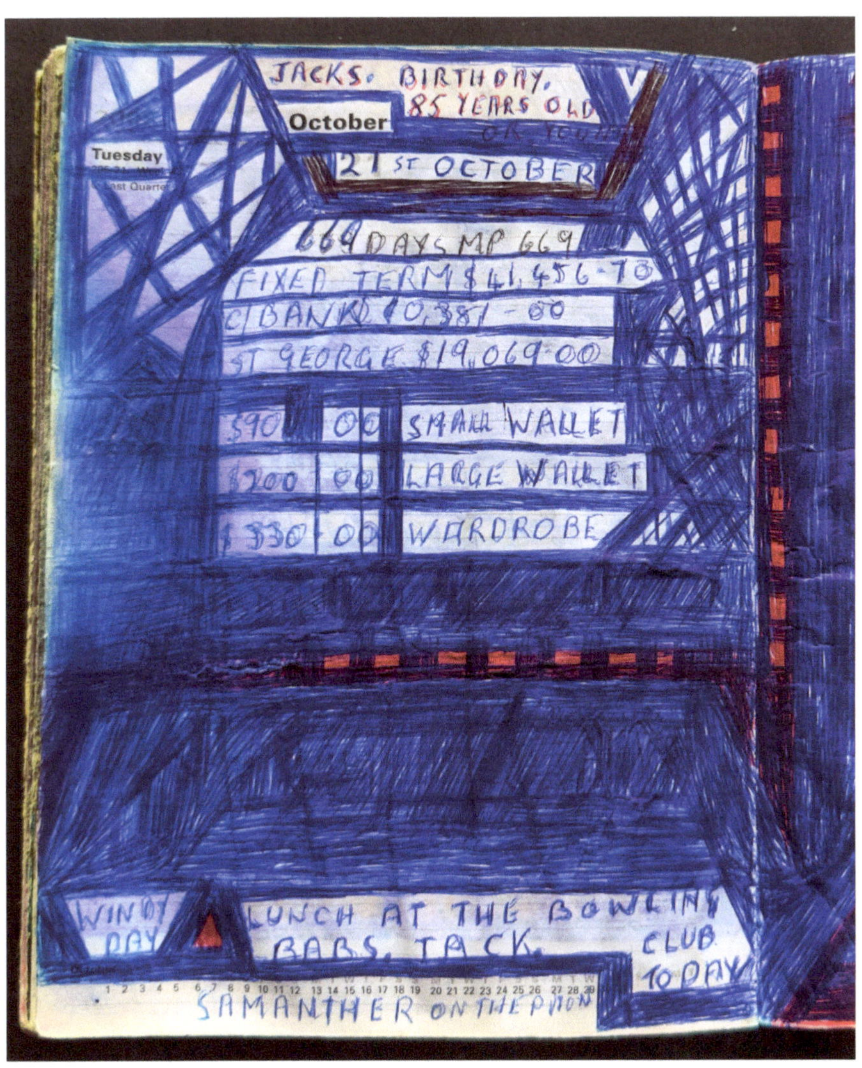
JACKS. BIRTHDAY.
85 YEARS OLD
October
Tuesday
Last Quarter
21ST OCTOBER
669 DAYS MP 669
FIXED TERM $41,456·70
C/BANK $10,381 - 00
ST GEORGE $19,069·00
$90   00   SMALL WALLET
$200   00   LARGE WALLET
$330   00   WARDROBE
WINDY DAY
LUNCH AT THE BOWLING CLUB
BABS, JACK.
TODAY
SAMANTHER ON THE PHON

December 28th

The residents in the villa block where Babs and Jack lived looked after each other. Babs is apparently the designated person with responsibility to take their own and their neighbour Lucy's bin down to the kerb.

Babs has apparently asked Jack to wash up after the washing machine stops. She definitely made an effort to help Jack to be able to keep track of what had to be done.

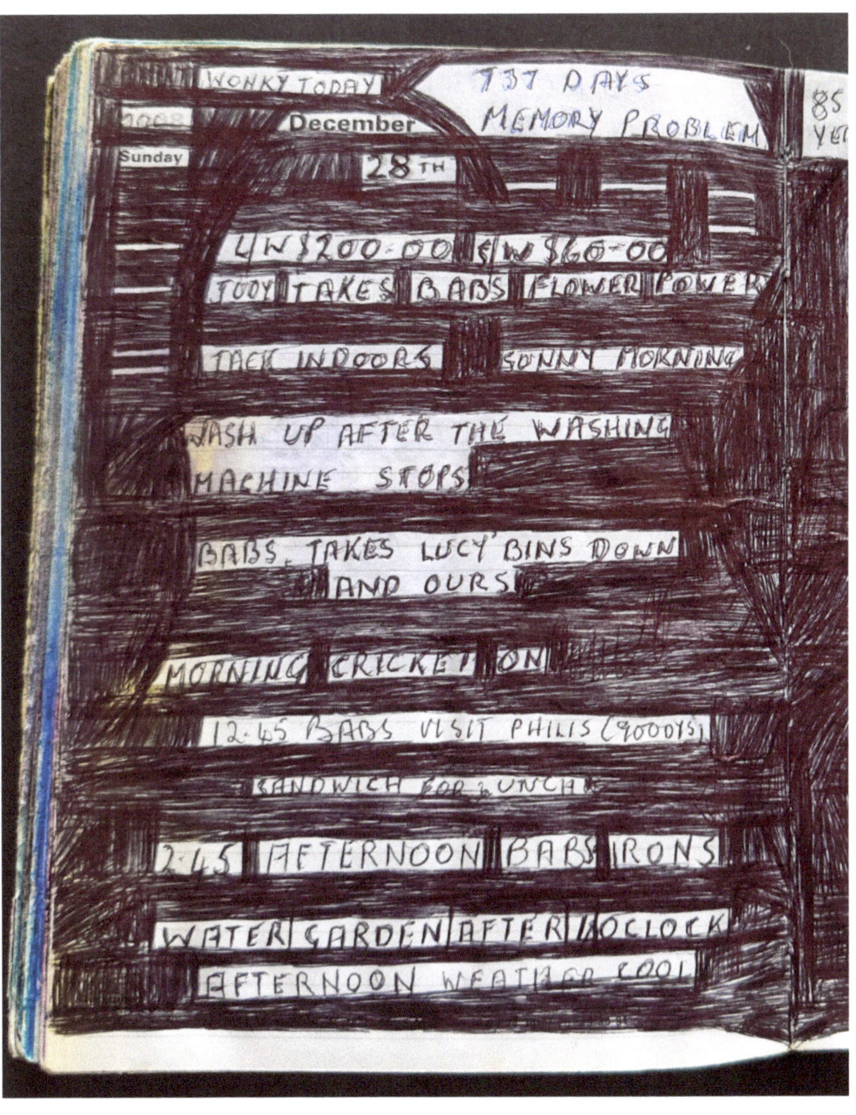
WONKY TODAY
737 DAYS
MEMORY PROBLEM
2008 December
85 YE
Sunday 28TH
4W $200·00 4W $60·00
TODY TAKES BABS FLOWER POWER
TACK INDOORS SUNNY MORNING
WASH UP AFTER THE WASHING
MACHINE STOPS
BABS TAKES LUCY BINS DOWN
AND OURS
MORNING CRICKET ON
12·45 BABS VISIT PHILIS (90DDYS)
SANDWICH FOR LUNCH
2·45 AFTERNOON BABS IRONS
WATER GARDEN AFTER 11OCLOCK
AFTERNOON WEATHER COOL

Chapter 4

2009

'I can't explain myself I'm afraid, sir,' said Alice, 'because I'm not myself, you see.'

January 5th

I noticed that the artwork is very dark as I looked through the 2009 diary. It's certainly darker than his previous diaries. Jack keeps recording his age and writes that he has a memory problem at the top of almost every page.

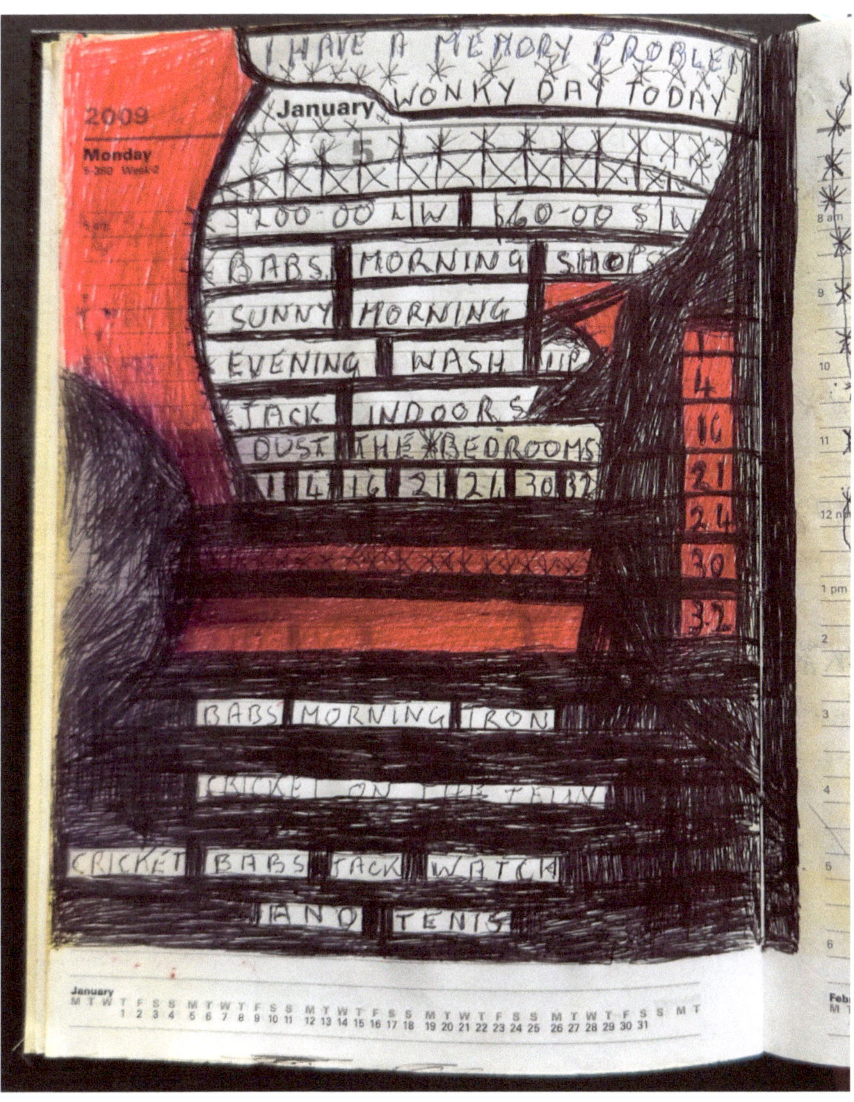
I HAVE A MEMORY PROBLEM
WONKY DAY TODAY
2009
Monday
5-280 Week-2
January
5
£200-00 L/W £60-00 S/W
BABS MORNING SHOPS
SUNNY MORNING
EVENING WASH UP
JACK INDOORS
DUST THE BEDROOMS
4 16 21 24 30 32
4
16
21
24
30
32
BABS MORNING IRON
CRICKET ON THE TELLY
CRICKET BABS JACK WATCH
JAND TENIS
January
M T W T F S S M T W T F S S M T W T F S S M T W T F S S M T W T F S S M T
1 2 3 4 5 6 7 8 9 10 11 12 13 14 15 16 17 18 19 20 21 22 23 24 25 26 27 28 29 30 31

January 31st & February 1st

Jack's still regularly recording his age as well as the Lotto and Pools results. He's noting that Babs went out to the bowling club yesterday, and that she went to visit Lucy the day before.

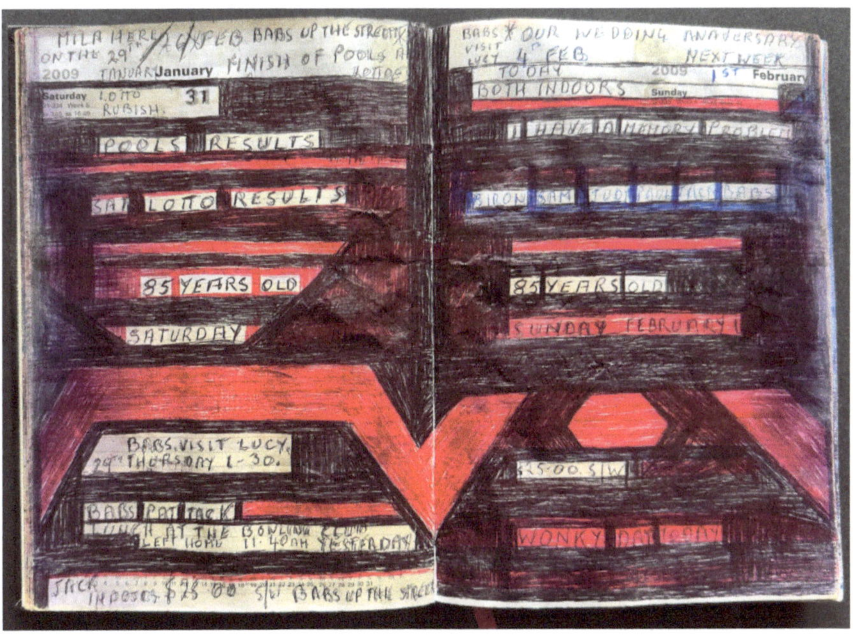
MILA HERE ON THE 29TH / 6/F FEB BABS UP THE STREET
FINISH OF POOLS A LOTTO
2009 JANUAR January
Saturday LOTTO 31
RUBISH.
POOLS RESULTS
SAT LOTTO RESULTS
85 YEARS OLD
SATURDAY
BABS.VISIT LUCY. 29TH THURSDAY 1-30.
BABS PAT TACK
LUNCH AT THE BOWLING CLUB
LEFT HOME 11.40AM YESTERDAY
JACK INDOORS $25.00 S/W BABS UP THE STREET
BABS * OUR WEDDING ANAVERSARY
VISIT LUCY 4 FEB NEXT WEEK
TODAY 2009 1ST February
BOTH INDOORS Sunday
I HAVE A MEMORY PROBLEM
BIRON SAM TUDI PAUL JACK BABS
85 YEARS OLD
SUNDAY FEBRUARY 1
$5.00 S/W
WONKY DOT TODAY

March 9th

Jack has added the names Babs, Eady, and Jeff to this entry. Jeff was their neighbour, so he was probably giving Babs and Edie a lift to the shops.

This was a time when Jack was able to say something like - 'A wonky day yesterday.' I say that because it means that his memory wasn't totally defunct. It also confirms that some days were better than others. Hopefully, this means that today is a better day, but if the darkness of the post is any indication, I suspect it may not have been.

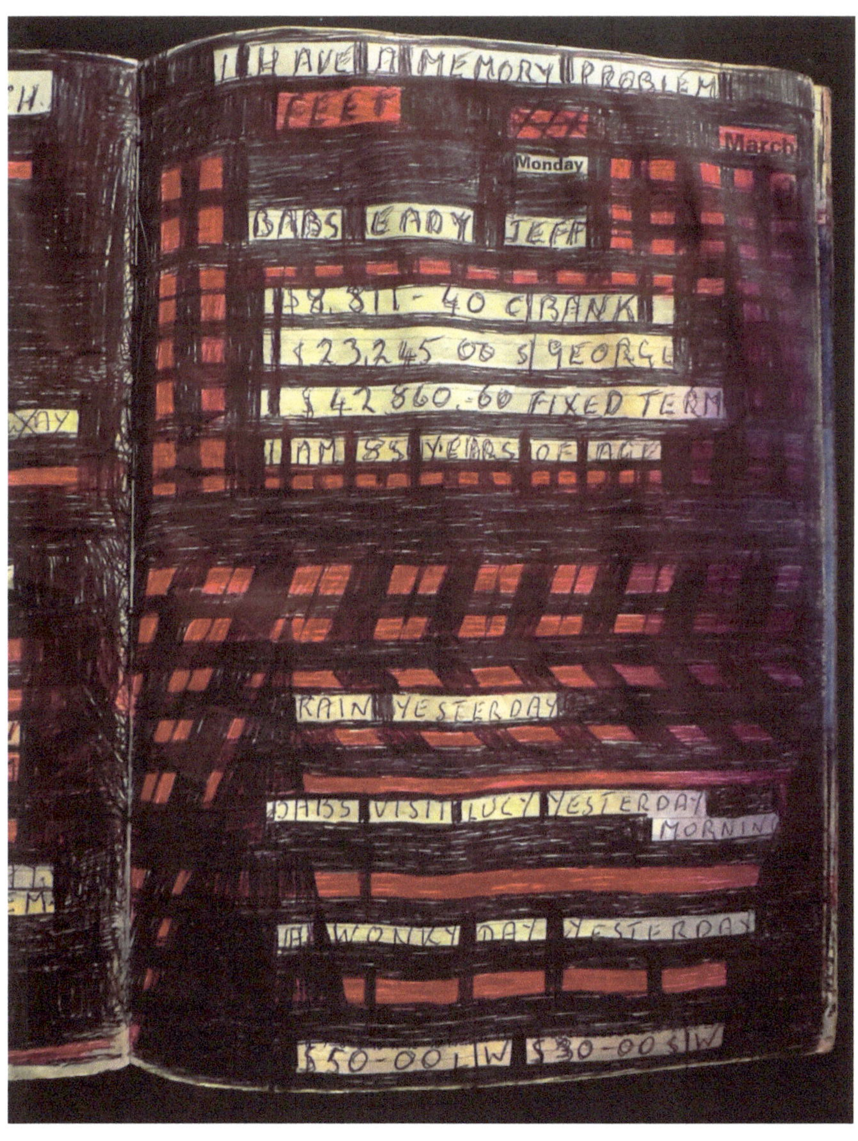
I HAVE A MEMORY PROBLEM
FEET
Monday
March
BABS EADY JEFF
$8.811 - 40 C/BANK
$23,245 00 S/ GEORGE
$42,860.60 FIXED TERM
I AM 85 YEARS OF AGE
RAIN YESTERDAY
BABS VISIT LUCY YESTERDAY
MORNING
A WONKY DAY YESTERDAY
$50-00 L/W $30-00 S/W

September 20th and 21st

It looks like Babs has bought Jack some new pens. He's really gone to town with colour here. I must say I'm really glad to see this, given the darkness of the earlier pages.

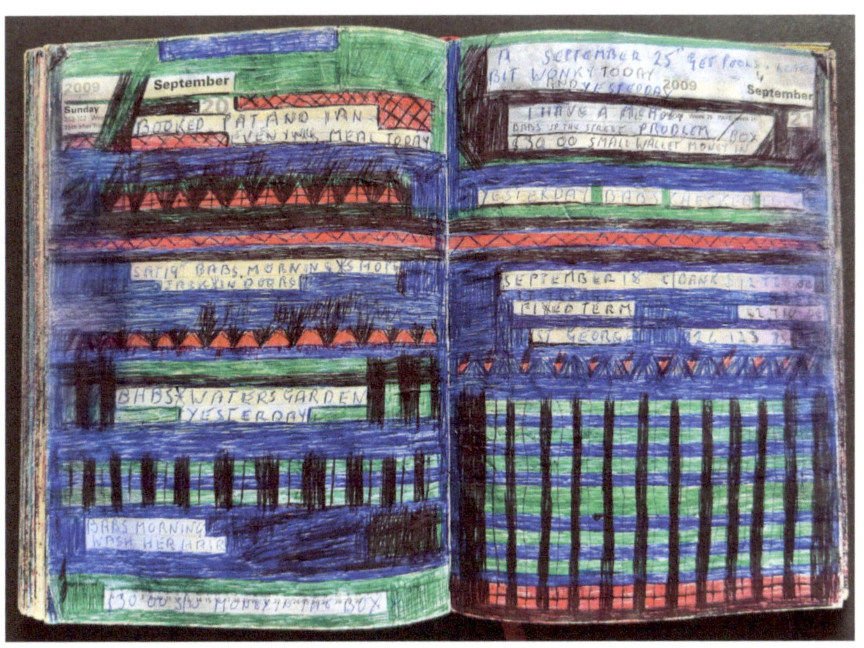
2009 September
Sunday 20
BOOKED PAT AND IAN EVENING MEAL TODAY
SAT 19" BABS MORNINGS SHOPPING FREE WINDOWS
BABS WATERS GARDEN YESTERDAY
BABS MORNING WASH HER HAIR
£30 00 S/W "MONEY IN THE "BOX
A SEPTEMBER 25" GET FOOLS
BIT WONKY TODAY
AND YESTERDAY 2009 September 21
I HAVE A MEMORY
BABS UP THE STREET PROBLEM BOX
£30 00 SMALL WALLET MONEY IN
YESTERDAY BABS CHECKED
SEPTEMBER 18 BANK
FIXED TERM
S/ GEORGE

September 30th

This is a fascinating entry. I looked at this page many times before I noticed that it is a mouth on the left-hand side of the drawing. Are there actually two faces?

What do you think?

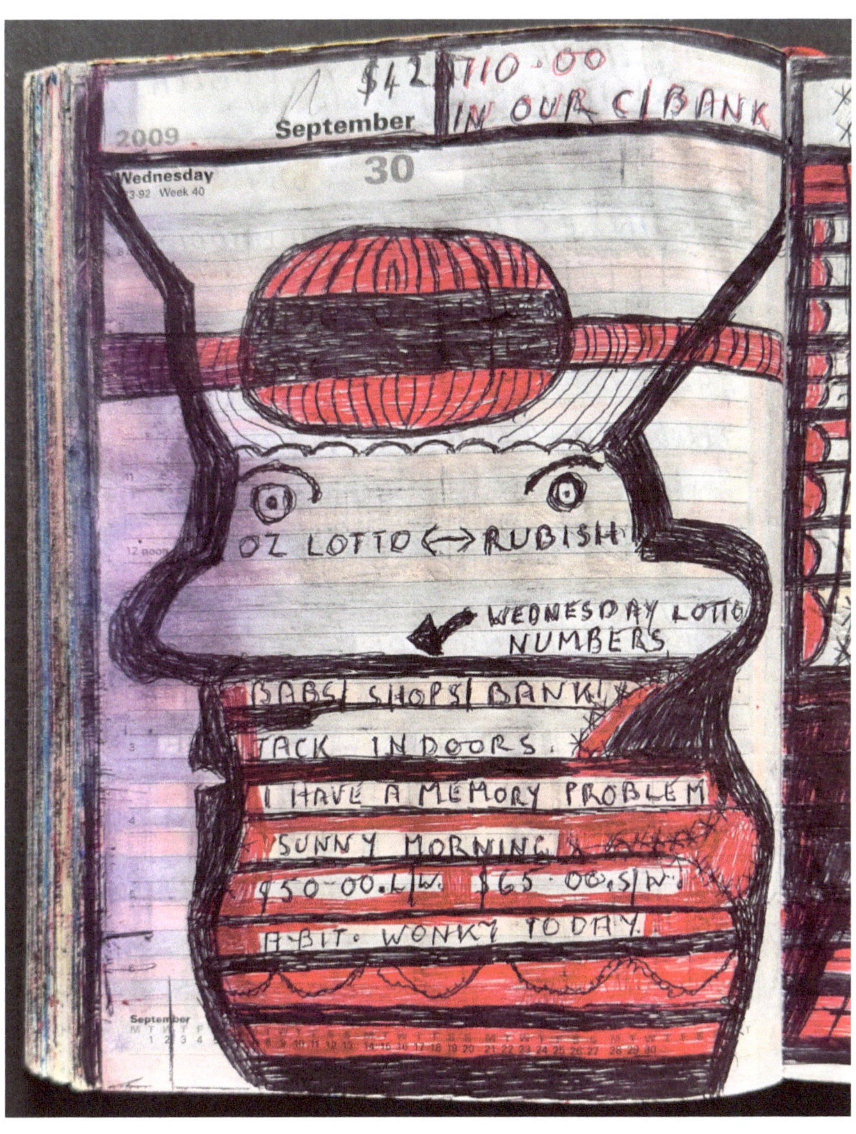
$42 710·00
IN OUR C/BANK
2009 September
30
Wednesday
3-92 Week 40
OZ LOTTO ⟷ RUBISH
WEDNESDAY LOTTO NUMBERS
BABS SHOPS BANK!
JACK INDOORS.
I HAVE A MEMORY PROBLEM
SUNNY MORNING.
$50·00 L.W. $65·00 S.W.
A BIT WONKY TODAY.

October 8th

Gordon was Babs's brother-in-law, who was very ill at this time. I feel like the barbed wire appearance and lack of colour in this entry could signify Jack's concern about his brother's state, as well as his own. I can only speculate of course, but I feel like something is going on here.

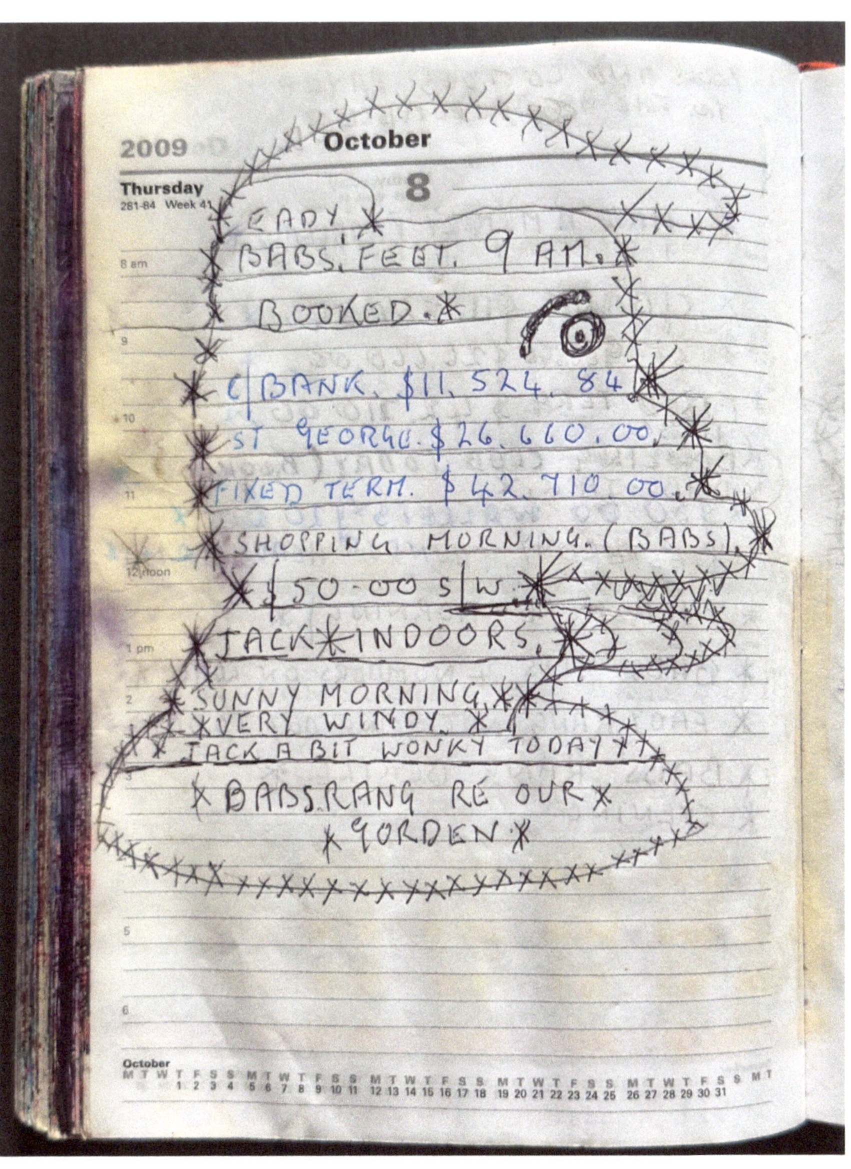
2009
October
Thursday
281-84 Week 41
8 am
9
10
11
12 noon
1 pm
2
3
4
5
6

EADY
BABS. FEET. 9 AM.
BOOKED.

C/BANK. $11,524,84
ST GEORGE. $26,660,00.
FIXED TERM. $42,710,00.
SHOPPING MORNING. (BABS).
$50.00 S/W.
JACK INDOORS.
SUNNY MORNING.
VERY WINDY.
JACK A BIT WONKY TODAY.
BABS. RANG RE OUR
GORDEN.

October
M T W T F S S M T W T F S S M T W T F S S M T W T F S S M T W T F S S M T
      1 2 3 4 5 6 7 8 9 10 11 12 13 14 15 16 17 18 19 20 21 22 23 24 25 26 27 28 29 30 31

Chapter 5

2010

'I'm sure those are not the right words,' said poor Alice

January 27th and 28th

It's a new year, and Jack has a bunch of new pens. There are some interesting patterns on these pages, and a heck of a lot of ink has been used.

Jack has noted that Babs is spending the morning up the street. I assume this means that Babs was shopping at Engadine.

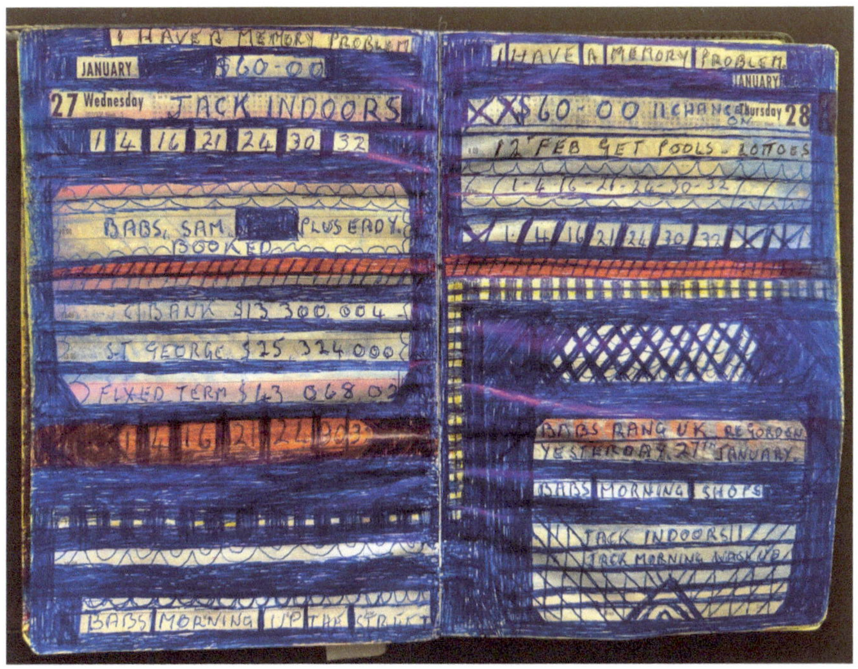
I HAVE A MEMORY PROBLEM
JANUARY $60-00
27 Wednesday JACK INDOORS
1 4 16 21 24 30 32
BABS, SAM PLUS EADY.
BOOKED
CITBANK $13 300 004
ST GEORGE $25 324 000
FIXED TERM $43 068 02
1 4 16 21 24 003
BABS MORNING UP THE STREET
I HAVE A MEMORY PROBLEM
JANUARY
$60-00 ILCHANCE Thursday 28
ON
12 FEB GET POOLS - LOTTOES
1 - 4 16 - 21 - 24 - 30 - 32
1 4 16 21 24 30 32
BABS RANG UK REJORDEN
YESTERDAY 27TH JANUARY.
BABS MORNING SHOTS
JACK INDOORS
JACK MORNING AROUND

February 10th and 11th

With Babs's help, Jack is still keeping track of their finances – hence he's written that all bills have been paid by 23 February. I imagine there would be some comfort in the fact that he feels like he's able to maintain some control, and a sense of comfort that they're OK financially.

I've looked at these pages many times, and it was years before I noticed that there are two profiled faces here – one on the left-hand page and the shaded one between the pages. My editor can't see the shaded one for the life of her. Can you see it – or is it just me?

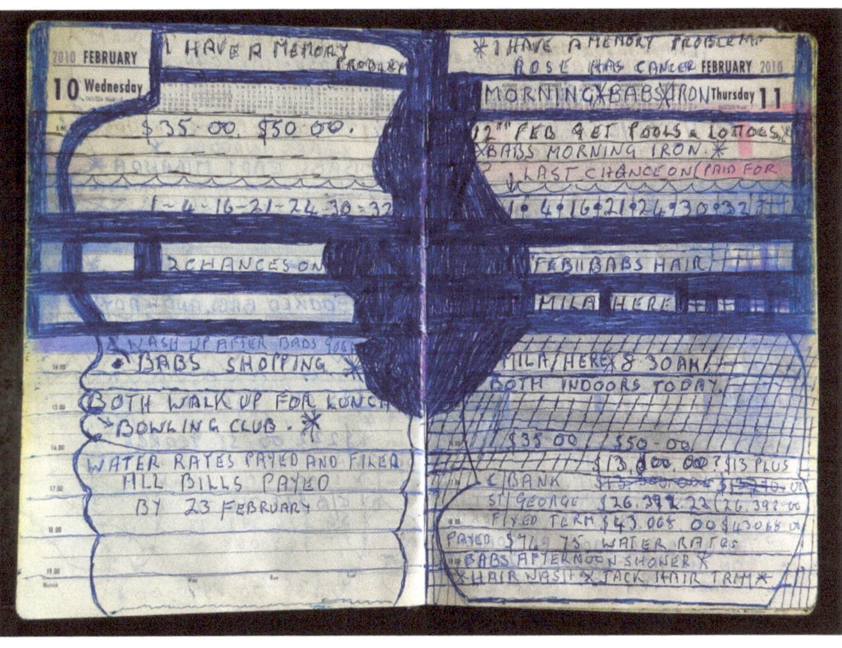
2010 FEBRUARY
10 Wednesday
I HAVE A MEMORY PROBLEM
$35.00. $50.00.
1 ~ 4 ~ 16 ~ 21 ~ 24 ~ 30 ~ 32
2 CHANCES ON
WASH UP AFTER BABS
BABS SHOPPING
BOTH WALK UP FOR LUNCH
BOWLING CLUB.
WATER RATES PAYED AND FILED
ALL BILLS PAYED
BY 23 FEBRUARY
* I HAVE A MEMORY PROBLEM
ROSE HAS CANCER FEBRUARY 2010
MORNING BABS IRON Thursday 11
12TH FEB GET POOLS & LOTTOES
BABS MORNING IRON.
LAST CHANCE ON (PAID FOR
1 · 4 · 16 · 21 · 24 · 30 · 32
FEB11 BABS HAIR
MILA HERE
MILA/HERE 8 30AM
BOTH INDOORS TODAY.
$35 00 $50 - 00
$13,000.00 ? $13 PLUS
C BANK
ST GEORGE $26.392.22 (26.392.00
FIXED TERM $43.068 00 $43068 00
PAYED $76.75 WATER RATES
BABS AFTERNOON SHOWER
HAIR WASH & JACK HAIR TRIM *

April 2nd

Babs must have been very tired. I say that because it wasn't a habit of hers to take morning and afternoon naps. I love that it's a cheeky-looking pic here! This suits Jack's nature. He was a cheeky, fun-loving character at his core.

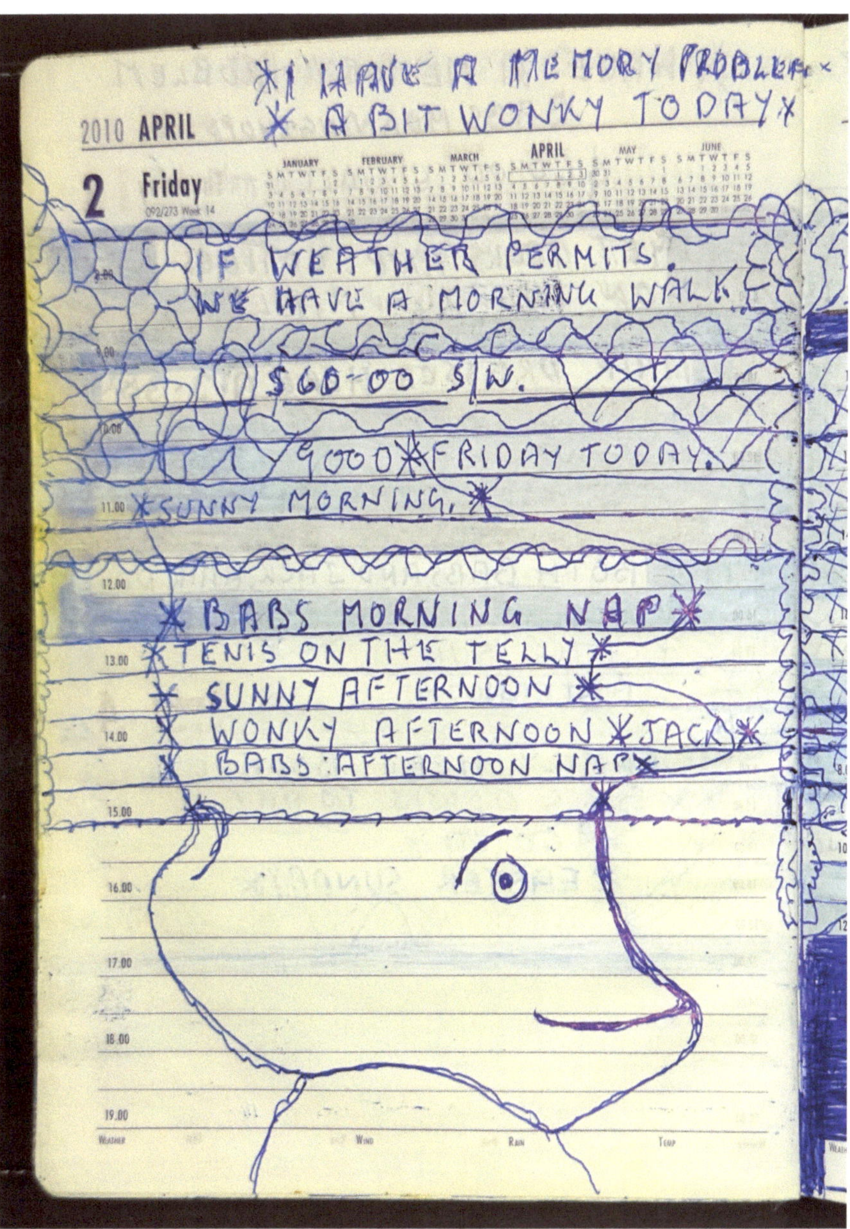
★ I HAVE A MEMORY PROBLEM ×
★ A BIT WONKY TODAY×
2010 APRIL
2 Friday
092/273 Week 14
IF WEATHER PERMITS.
WE HAVE A MORNING WALK.
$60-00 S/W.
9:00 ★ FRIDAY TODAY.
★ SUNNY MORNING. ★
★ BABS MORNING NAP ★
★ TENIS ON THE TELLY ★
★ SUNNY AFTERNOON ★
WONKY AFTERNOON ★ JACK ★
★ BABS AFTERNOON NAP ★

April 14^(th) and 15^(th)

There are lots of little squares on these pages. Needless to say, a whole lot of ink was used. I like the little smiley face at the top of April 14^(th) because it balances out the darkness of these pages a bit.

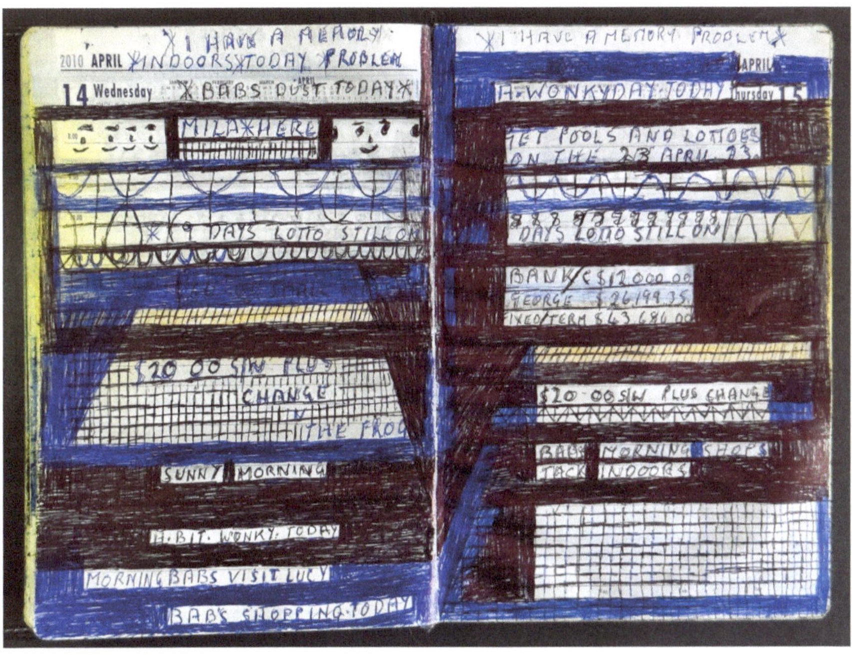
I HAVE A MEMORY PROBLEM
2010 APRIL *INDOORS*TODAY *PROBLEM
14 Wednesday *BABS DUST TODAY*
MILA*HERE
*9 DAYS LOTTO STILL ON
$20.00 S/W PLUS
CHANGE
THE FROG
SUNNY MORNING
H.BIT.WONKY.TODAY
MORNING BABS VISIT LUCY
BABS SHOPPING TODAY
I HAVE A MEMORY PROBLEM
APRIL
H.WONKYDAY TODAY Thursday 15
GET POOLS AND LOTTOES
ON THE 23 APRIL 23
888 88888888
8 DAYS LOTTO STILL ON
BANK/ €$12,000.00
GEORGE $26,199.35
FIXED/TERM $43,680.00
$20.00 S/W PLUS CHANGE
BABS MORNING SHOPS
TACK INDOORS

August 19th

There are lots of swirly patterns on this page, and what could be a self-portrait. I think the face is a happy one, but I can't be sure.

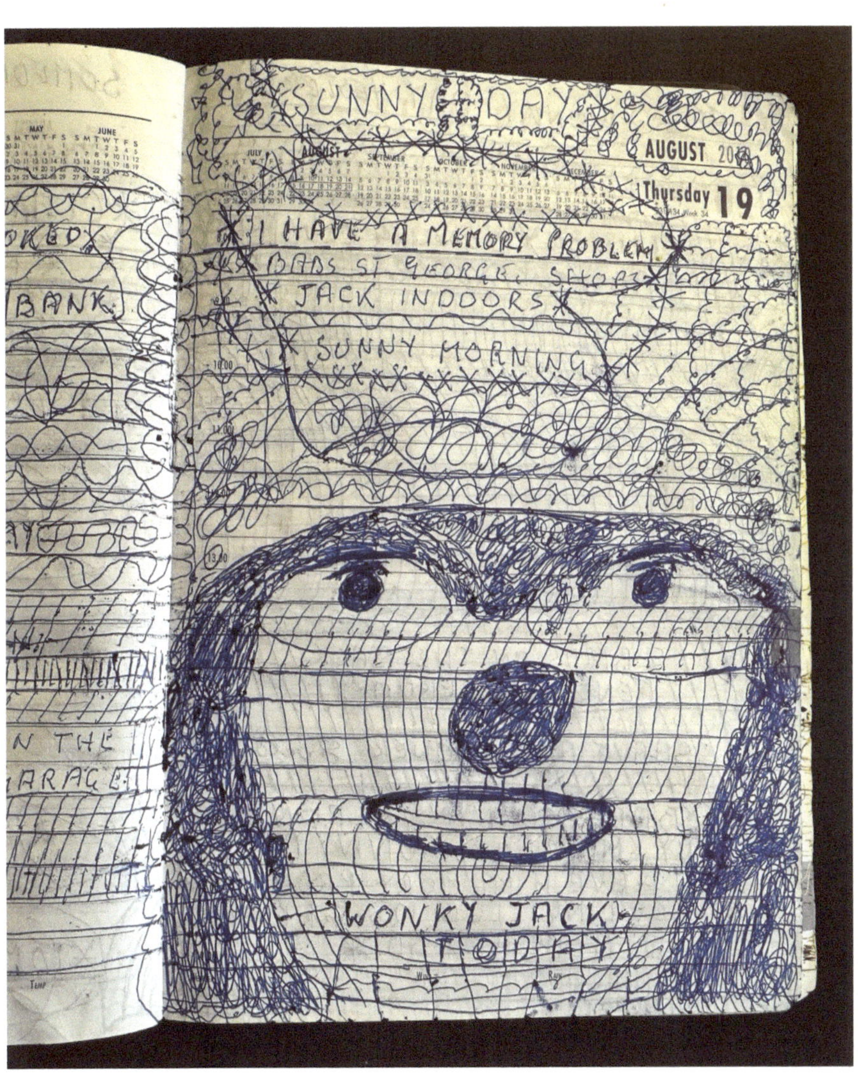
SUNNY DAY
AUGUST 2010
Thursday 19
I HAVE A MEMORY PROBLEM
BADS ST GEORGE. SHOPS
JACK INDOORS
SUNNY MORNING
WONKY JACK
TODAY

October 14th

I think Jack was looking forward to his salmon sandwich once Babs and Edie got back from the shops.

I love that Jack's comparing his age to Cliff Richard's. I'm not sure what the significance of the car in this image is.

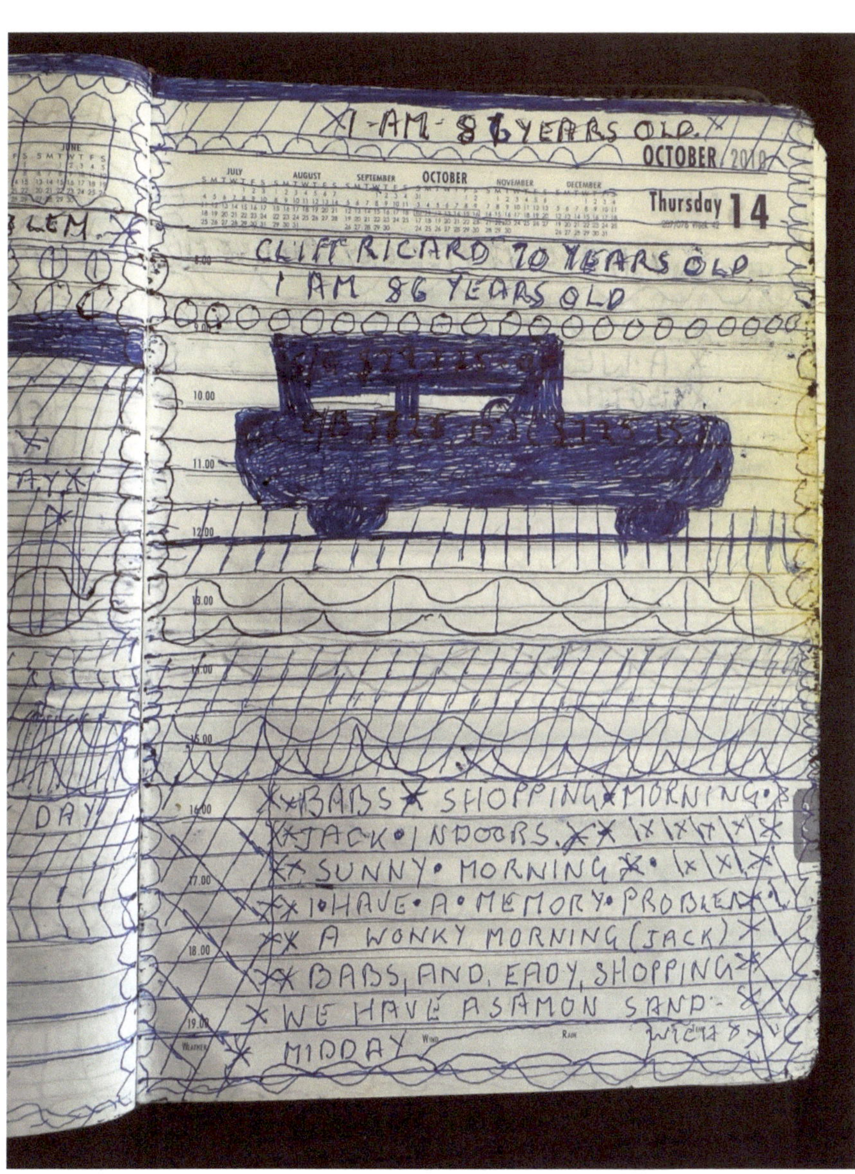
I·AM·86 YEARS OLD.
OCTOBER 2010
JULY AUGUST SEPTEMBER OCTOBER NOVEMBER DECEMBER
Thursday 14
CLIFF RICARD 70 YEARS OLD
I AM 86 YEARS OLD
BABS SHOPPING MORNING·
JACK·INDOORS.
SUNNY·MORNING
I·HAVE·A·MEMORY·PROBLEM
A WONKY MORNING (JACK)
BABS, AND, EADY, SHOPPING
WE HAVE A SAMON SAND-
MIDDAY WICH
WIND RAIN WEATHER

Chapter 6

2011

'So you think you're changed, do you?' said the Caterpillar.

'I'm afraid I am, sir,' said Alice; 'I can't remember things as I used.'

January 29th

There's a lot of barbed wire-like patterning on the next page, and no colour has been used. I went to Google to get a view on what this might mean. Apparently, barbed wire can symbolise feelings of oppression or confinement. I guess that makes sense, but I'm conscious of not reading too much into things like this because Jack is the only one who would have known for sure.

February 2011
March 2011
April 2011

January
WEEK 4

029/336 Saturday **29**

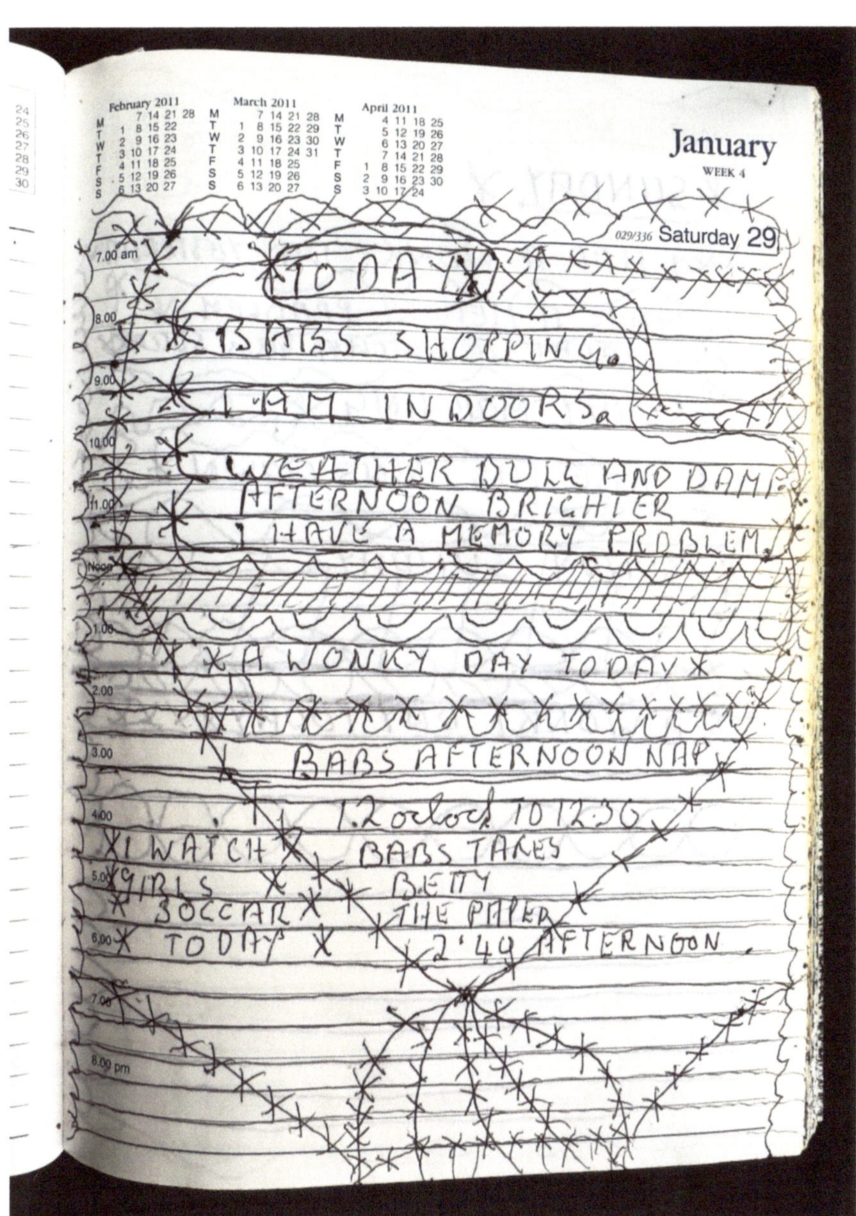

February 4th

I'm guessing Babs has reminded Jack that today is their wedding anniversary. Again, there is no colour used in this image.

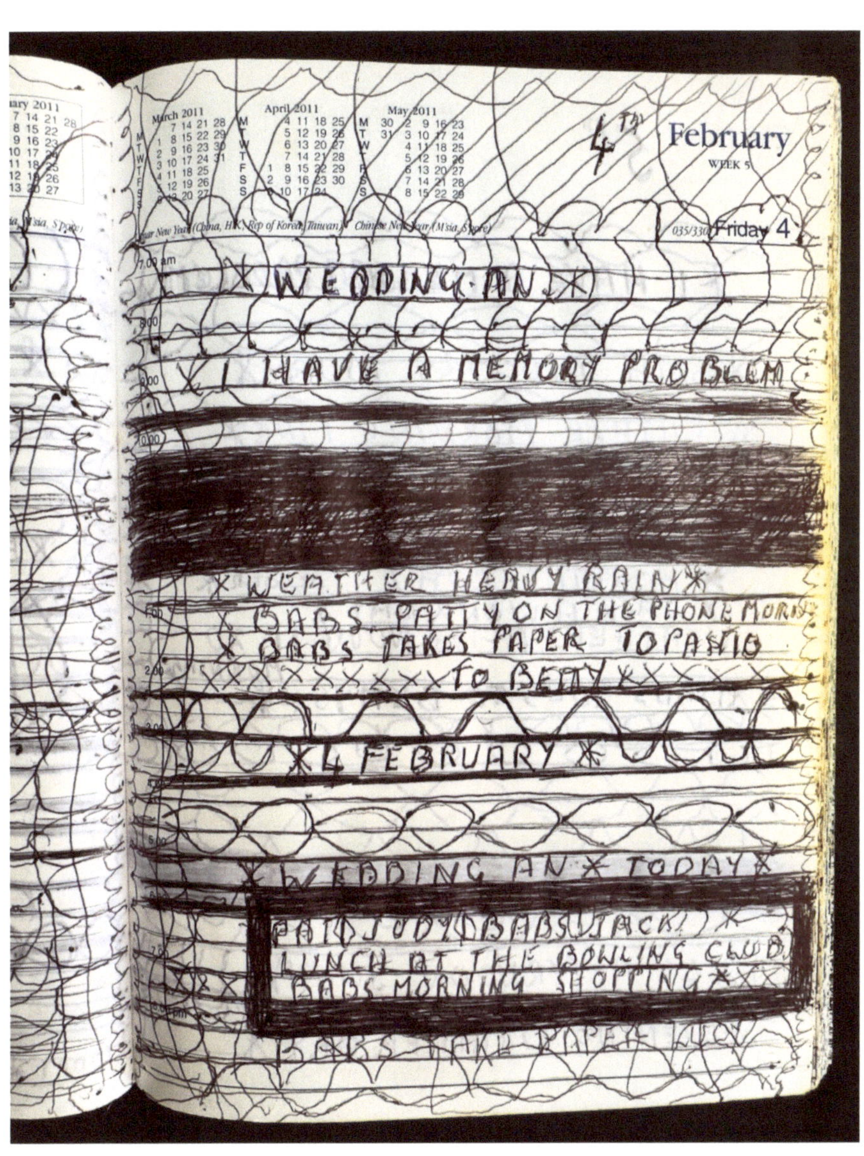
February
WEEK 5
Friday 4
* WEDDING AN *
I HAVE A MEMORY PROBLEM
* WEATHER HEAVY RAIN *
BABS. PATTY ON THE PHONE MORNS
* BABS TAKES PAPER TO PATIO
to BETTY
* 4 FEBRUARY *
* WEDDING AN * TODAY *
PAID JUDY * BABS * JACK *
LUNCH AT THE BOWLING CLUB
BABS MORNING SHOPPING
BABS TAKES PAPER

June 13th

'4 chances to win' says Jack the optimist. The Queen got a mention on this page as well. Jack wasn't a huge royalist, but he was rather fond of the Queen.

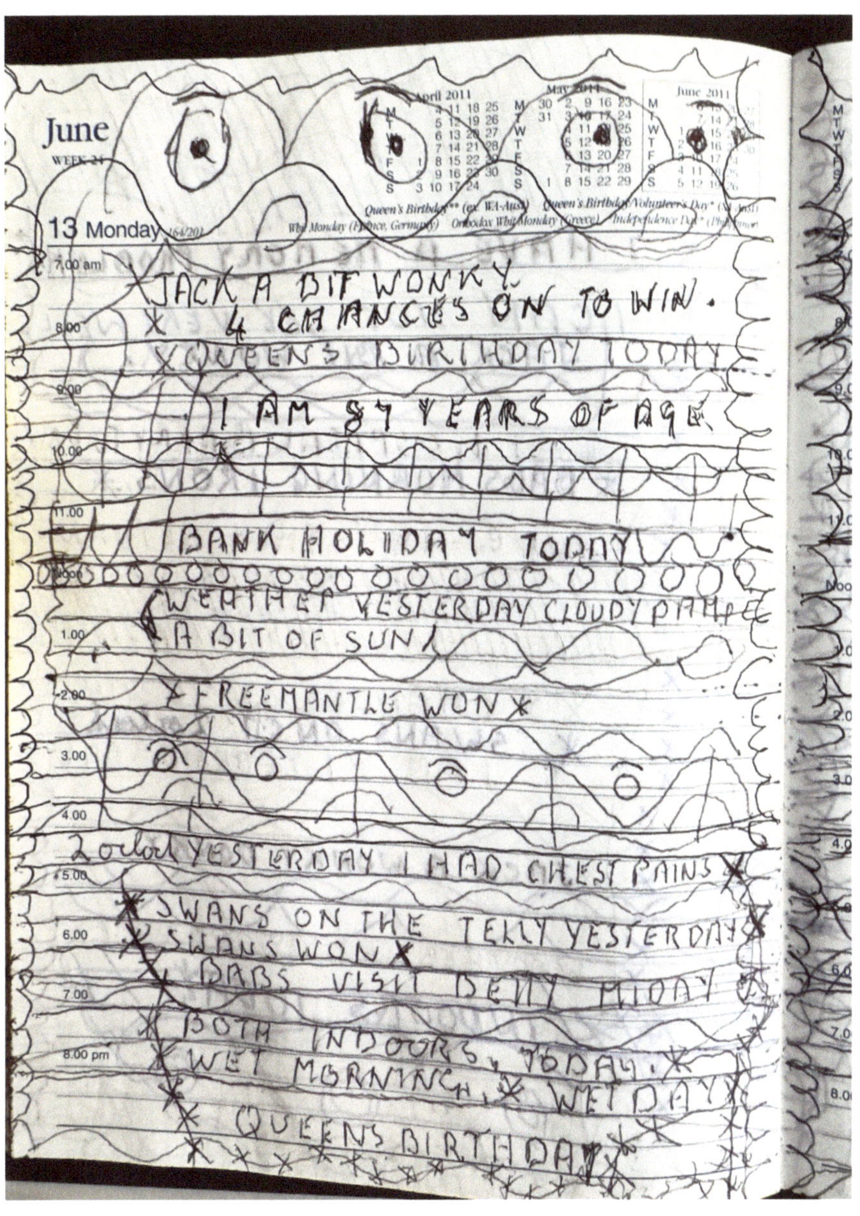
June
WEEK 24
13 Monday 164/201

JACK A BIT WONKY.
4 CHANCES ON TO WIN.
QUEENS BIRTHDAY TODAY
I AM 87 YEARS OF AGE.
BANK HOLIDAY TODAY
WEATHER YESTERDAY CLOUDY P.M.
A BIT OF SUN.
FREEMANTLE WON
2 oclock YESTERDAY I HAD CHEST PAINS
SWANS ON THE TELLY YESTERDAY
SWANS WON
BABS VISIT DENTY FRIDAY
BOTH INDOORS TODAY.
WET MORNING. WET DAY
QUEENS BIRTHDAY

September 27th

As it was with the previous few pages, there is a lot going on in this image. I think it's fair to say that Jack was having one of his happier days.

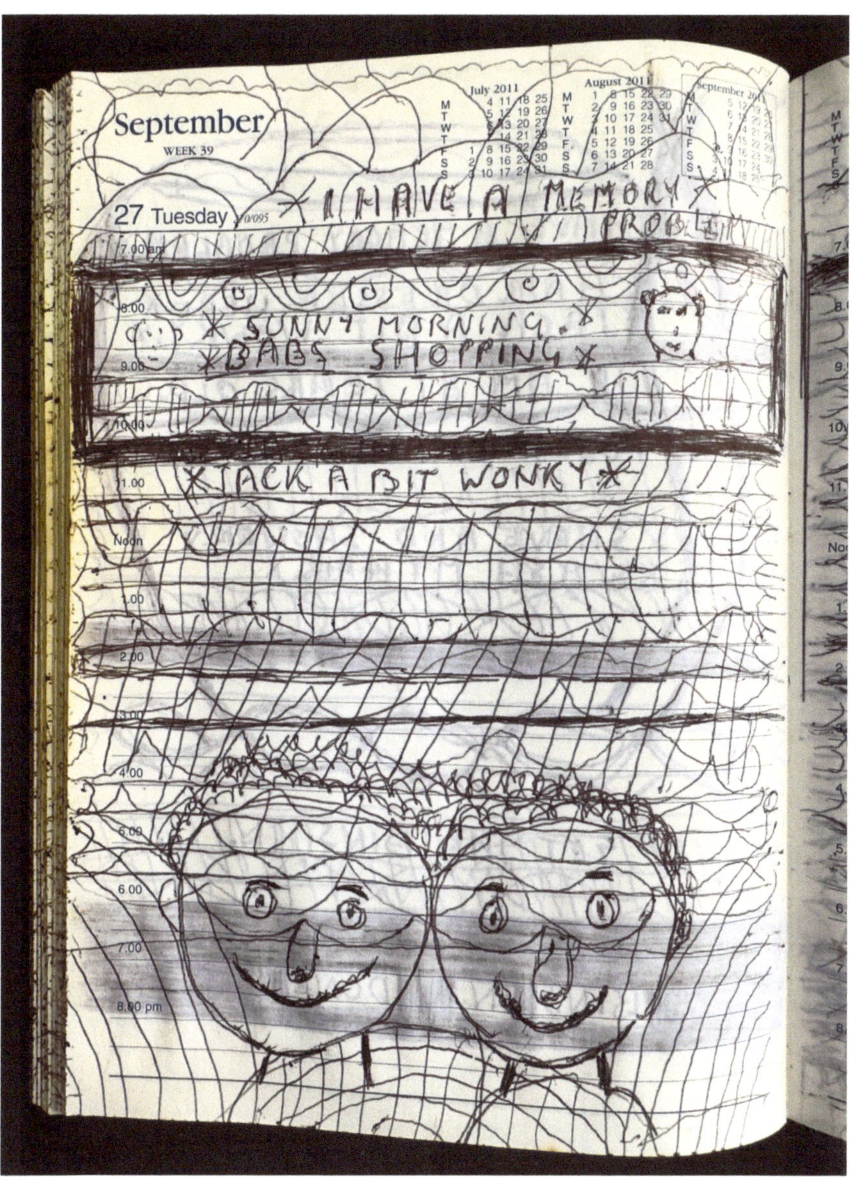
September
WEEK 39
27 Tuesday
July 2011
August 2011
September 2011
I HAVE A MEMORY PROBLEM
SUNNY MORNING
BABS SHOPPING
JACK A BIT WONKY

Chapter 7

2012

'What a curious feeling!' said Alice; 'I must be shutting up like a telescope.'

April 11th

Jack's diary entries are becoming less frequent, and it feels as if his writing is becoming more laboured.

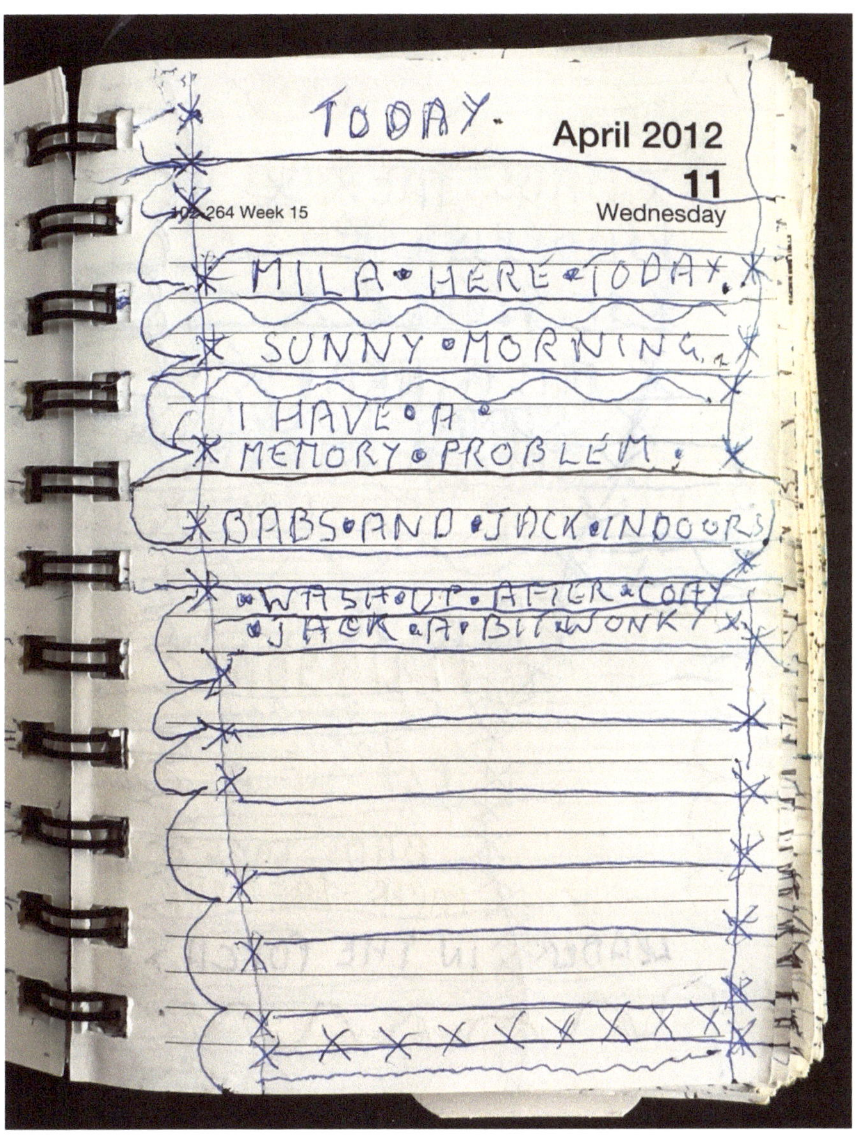
TODAY.
April 2012
11
Wednesday
102-264 Week 15
MILA • HERE • TODAY. •
SUNNY • MORNING.
I HAVE • A •
MEMORY • PROBLEM •
BABS • AND • JACK • INDOORS
• WASH UP • AFTER • COFY
• JACK • A • BIT • WONKY

April 12th

We teased Jack a bit, often saying, 'Are you a Wonky Donkey today, Dad?' He really liked the playfulness of that nickname and kind of took it on board.

The Leader is the local paper that Jack notes is on the porch, adding that Babs takes a copy to their neighbour, Betty.

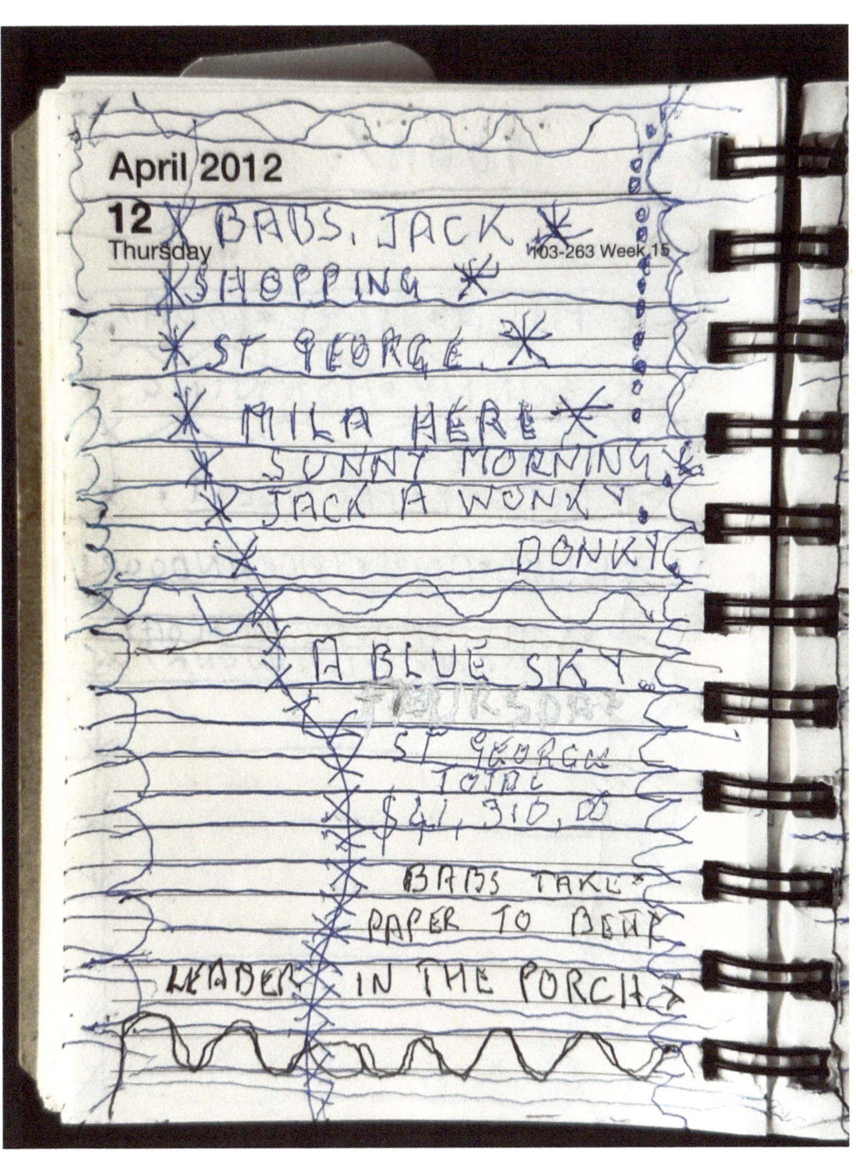
April 2012
12
Thursday
103-263 Week 15
BABS, JACK
SHOPPING
ST GEORGE.
MILA HERE
SUNNY MORNING
JACK A WONKY
DONKY
A BLUE SKY
THURSDAY
ST GEORGE
TOTAL
$41,310.00
BABS TAKE
PAPER TO DEBE
LEADER IN THE PORCH

April 18th

I'm guessing Babs has told Jack to write 'I wake up with Today' in his diary, and to answer the phone if it rings by saying those words in order to win the glittering prizes they were offering. *The Today Show* is a popular morning television show in Australia that's still running as I'm pulling this material together in 2025.

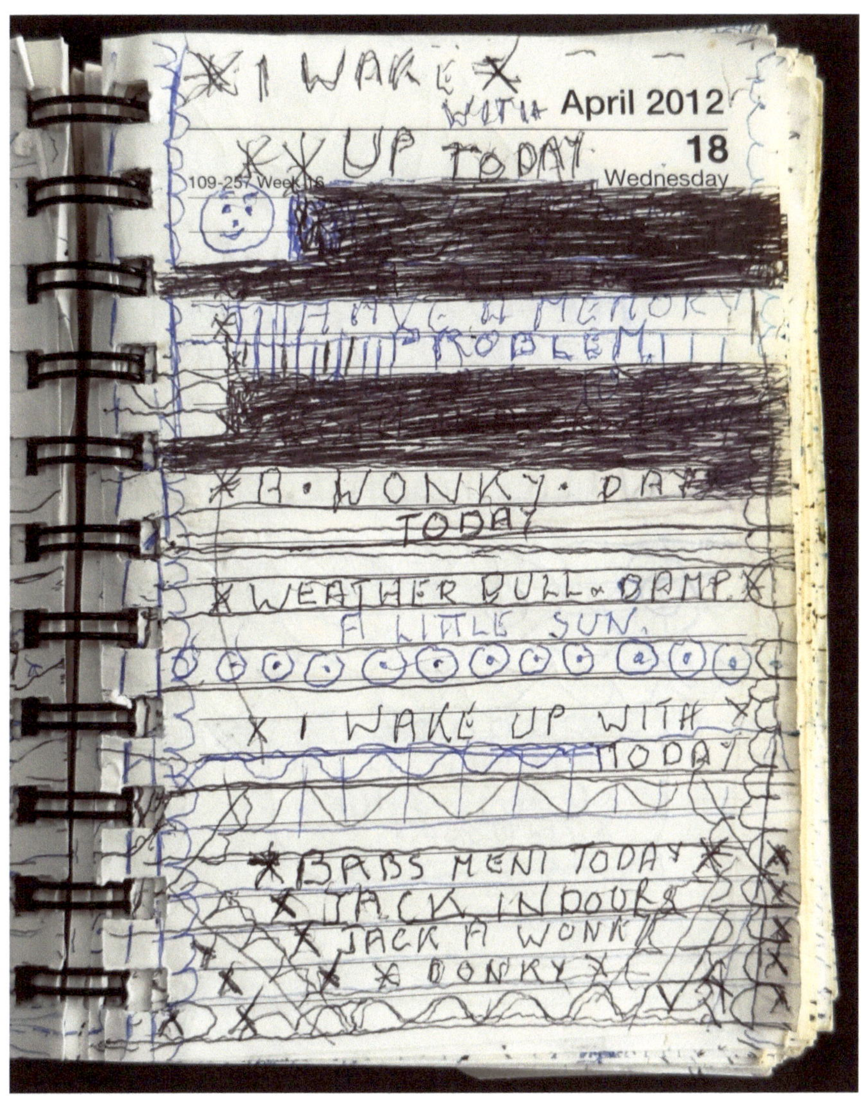
I WAKE
UP TODAY WITH
April 2012
18
Wednesday
109-257 Week 16
HAVE A MEMORY
PROBLEM
A WONKY DAY
TODAY
WEATHER DULL & DAMP
A LITTLE SUN.
I WAKE UP WITH
TODAY
BRBS MEN! TODAY
JACK INDOORS
JACK A WONKY
DONKY

April 21st

Dad was a bit of a fan of the football. His favourite team, called The Swans, must have been playing. Overall, it feels like Jack was having a good day, especially with something he enjoyed watching on the telly.

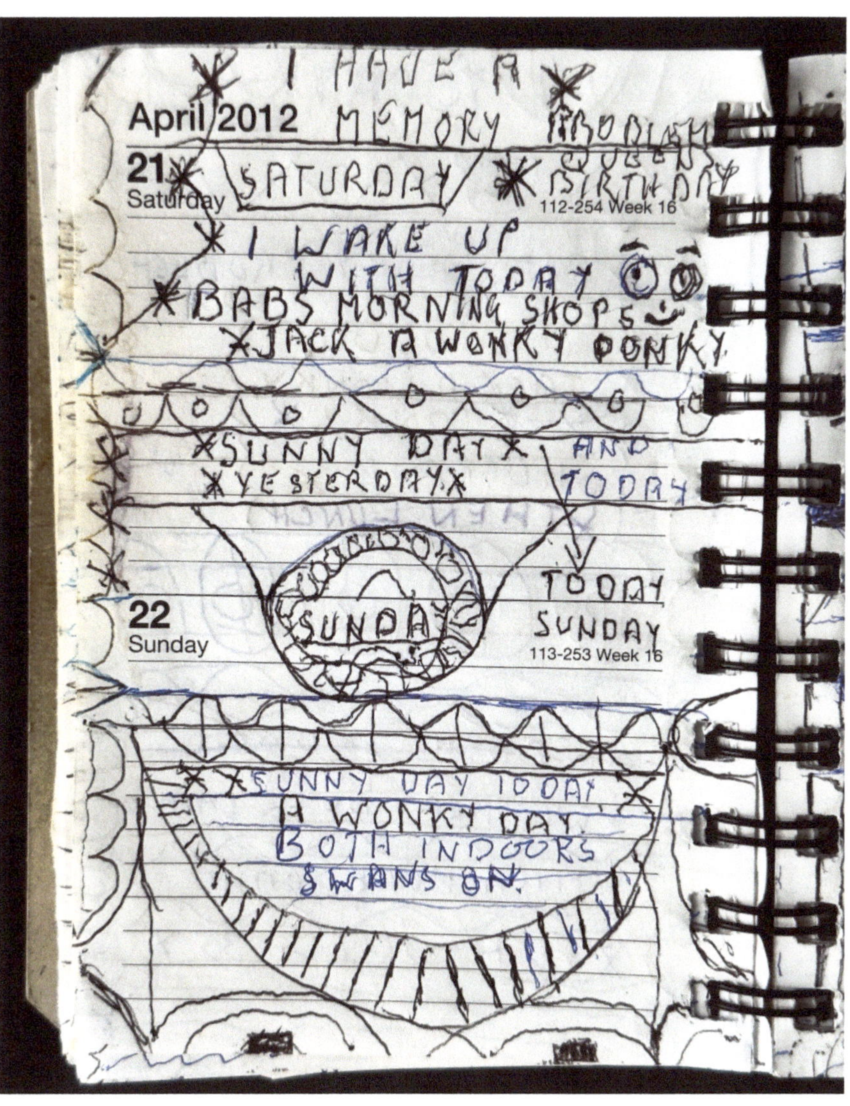
April 2012
I HAVE A MEMORY PROBLEM
21 SATURDAY QUEEN BIRTHDAY
Saturday
112-254 Week 16
I WAKE UP WITH TODAY
BABS MORNING SHOPS
JACK A WONKY DONKY
SUNNY DAY AND
YESTERDAY TODAY
TODAY
22 SUNDA SUNDAY
Sunday
113-253 Week 16
SUNNY DAY TODAY
A WONKY DAY
BOTH INDOORS
SWANS ON.

May 16th

I feel like Babs probably really needed that potter in the garden that Jack mentions. I wonder whether, for some reason, Jack was trying to focus on where Babs was, or maybe it just made him happy to know that she was out in the garden pottering around and enjoying herself.

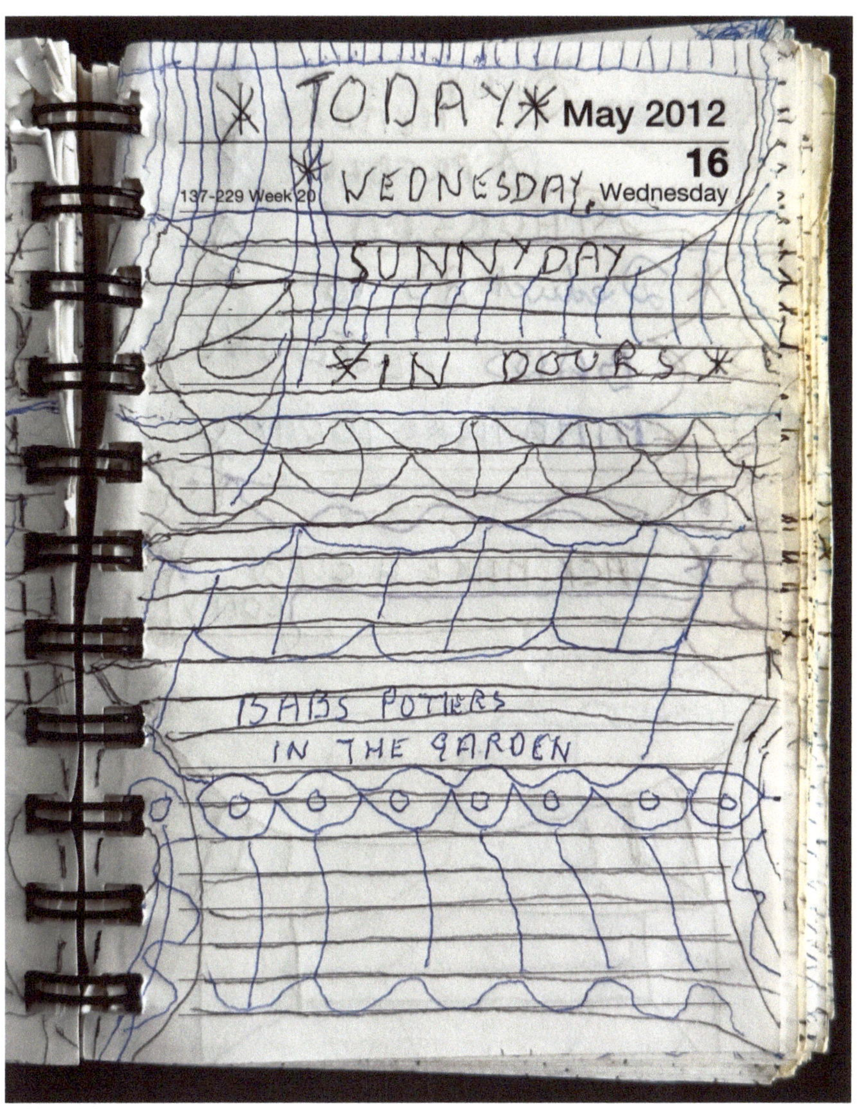
* TODAY * May 2012
137-229 Week 20
* WEDNESDAY,
16
Wednesday
SUNNY DAY
* IN DOORS *
ISABS POTIERS
IN THE GARDEN

May 18th

My sister Judy has taken Babs to her doctor's appointment. Babs has probably reminded Jack to have a shower and shampoo his hair. No lotto numbers are recorded on this day, but Jack has noted that it was a sunny day.

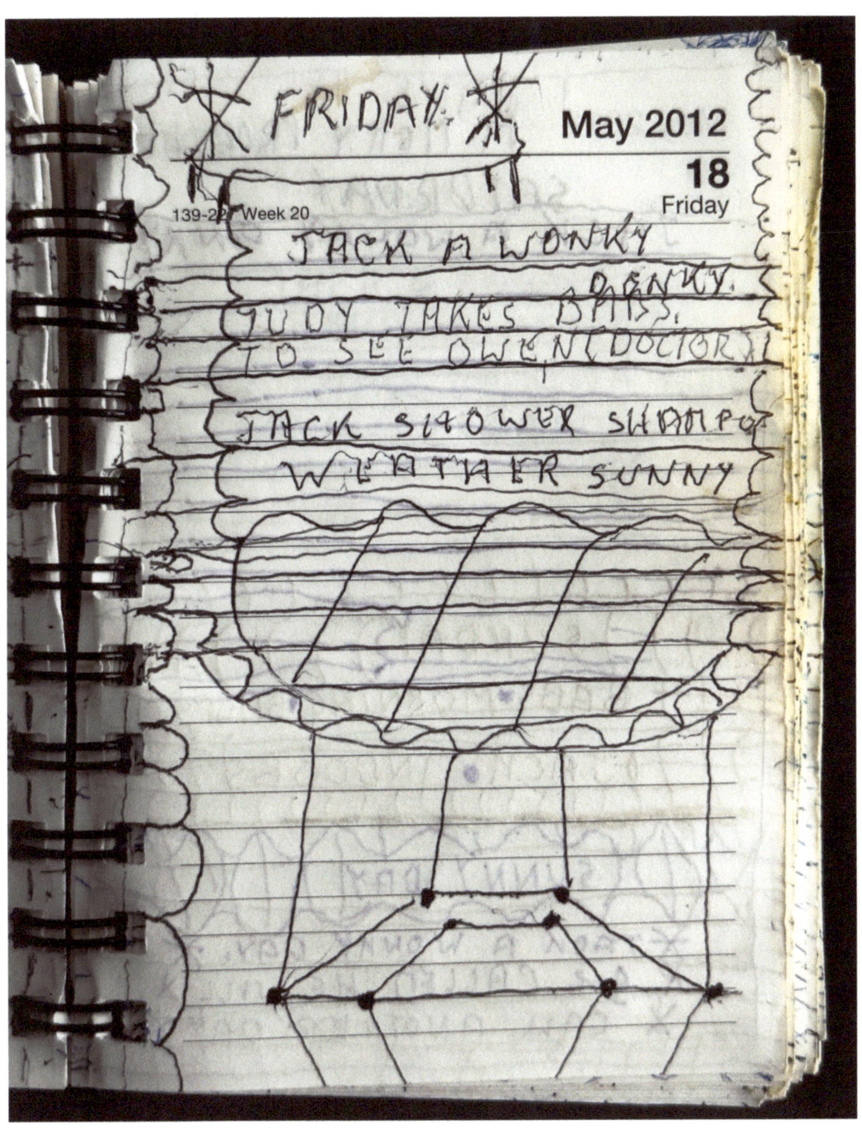
FRIDAY.
May 2012
18
Friday
139-22 Week 20
JACK A WONKY
DONKY.
JUDY TAKES DADS.
TO SEE OWEN(DOCTOR).
JACK SHOWER SHAMPO
WEATHER SUNNY

May 26th

It's hard to miss the tone of this entry. The barbed wire effect seems to suggest Jack is feeling trapped. While I always tell people that Jack's journey with dementia isn't necessarily a sad story, I have to say that for me, this is one of the more unsettling entries in the 7 diaries Jack left as his legacy.

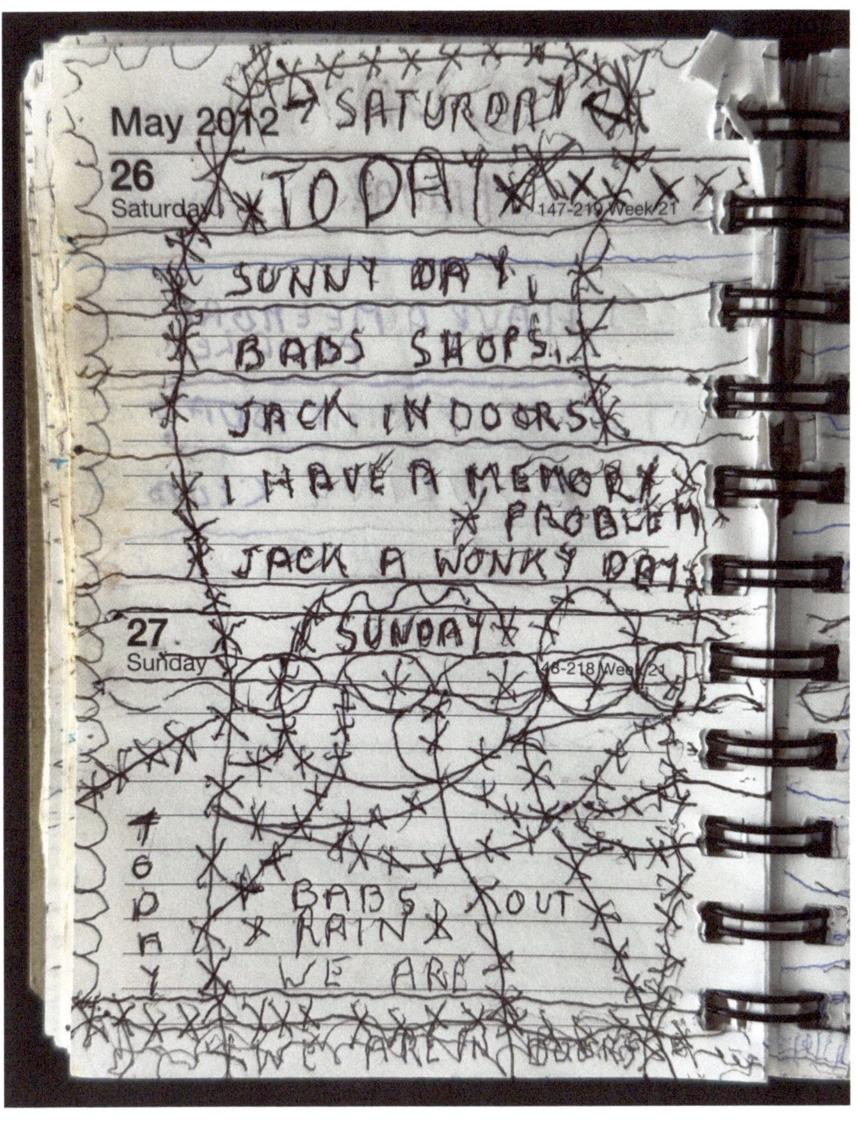
May 2012
26 Saturday
147-219 Week 21
→ SATURDAY ←
TODAY
SUNNY DAY
BABS SHOPS.
JACK INDOORS
I HAVE A MEMORY PROBLEM
JACK A WONKY DAY
27 Sunday
46-218 Week 21
SUNDAY
TODAY
BABS OUT
RAIN
WE ARE
WE ARE IN DOORS

June 15th

This appears to be a happier day for Jack. There's a smiley face and some fun doodles included.

You might not be able to discern the words on the 4th line. They are – 'With Paty'. I'm the Paty he's talking about here. We ventured out for lunch at the bowling club today, as we did from time to time. He used to love outings like these.

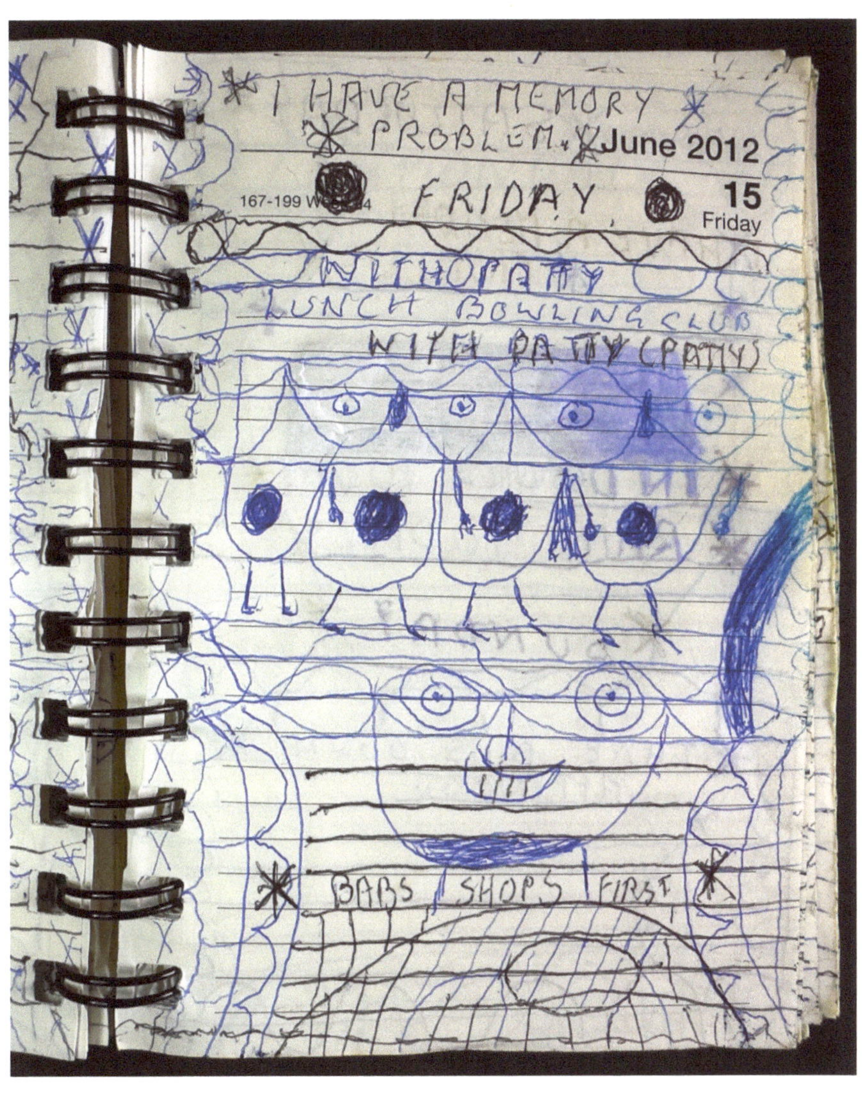
I HAVE A MEMORY PROBLEM
PROBLEM
June 2012
167-199 Week 24
FRIDAY
15
Friday
WITH PATTY
LUNCH BOWLING CLUB
WITH PATTY (PATTY)
BABS SHOPS FIRST

July 10th

Jack's diary entries are becoming, in his words, 'Wonky'. There has been a heck of a lot of back and forth with the blue pen on the opposite page, that's for sure!

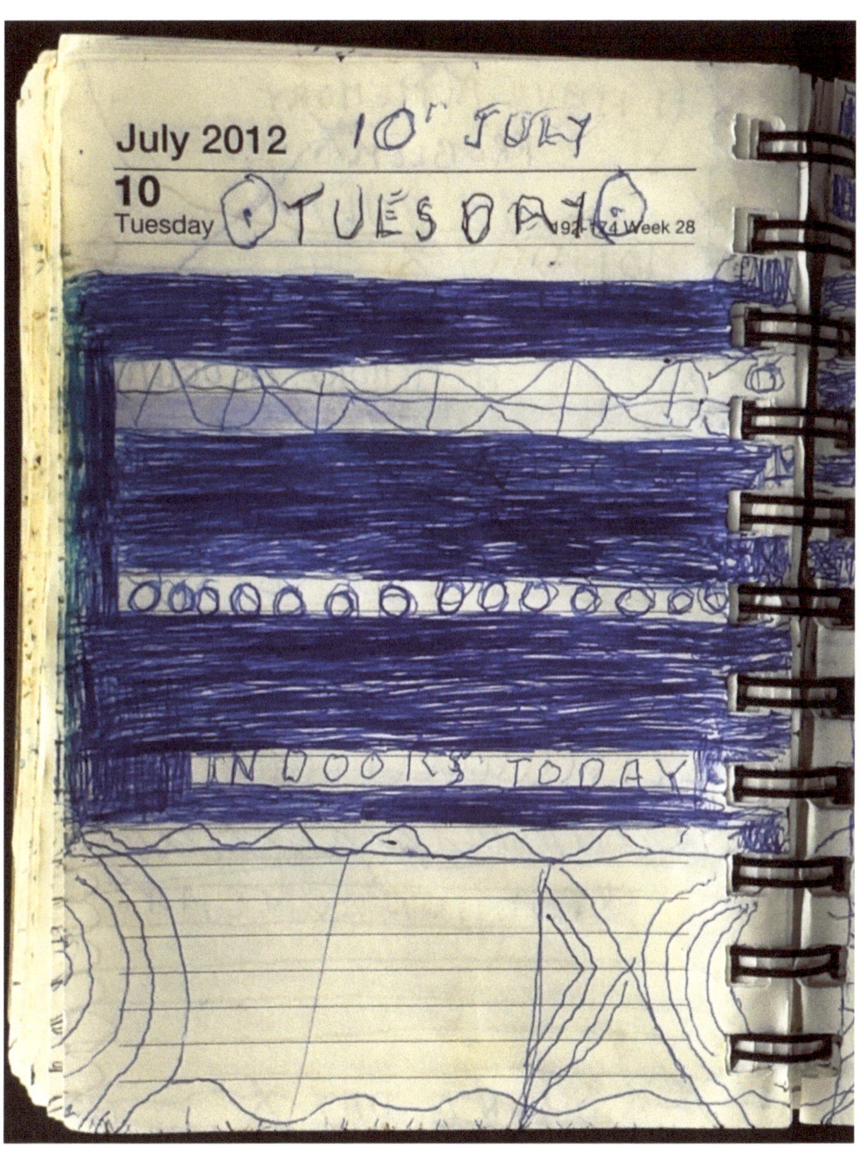
July 2012
10
Tuesday
10TH JULY
TUESDAY
192-174 Week 28
INDOORS TODAY

July 11th

Babs must have been getting a lift to somewhere while Jack was staying home – indoors, as he says. It's quite likely that Babs was going to do some shopping.

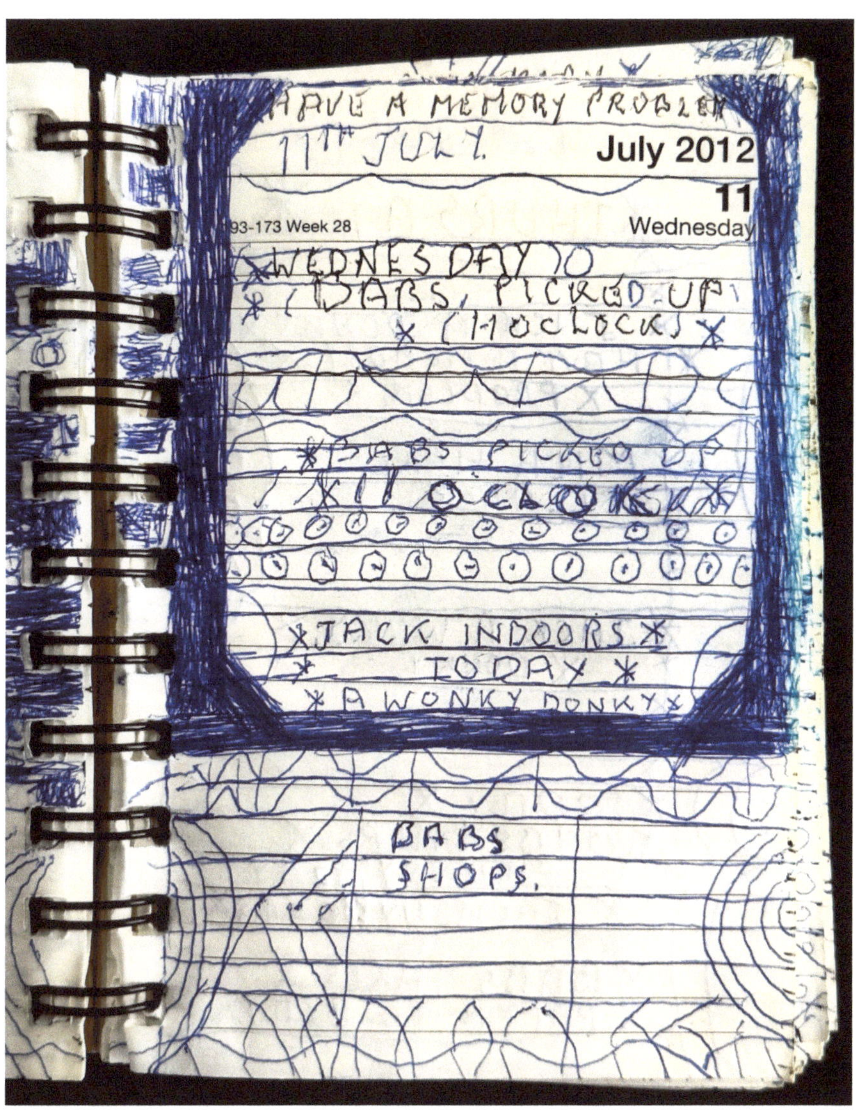
HAVE A MEMORY PROBLEM
11TH JULY.
July 2012
193-173 Week 28
11
Wednesday
WEDNESDAY
(BABS, PICKED UP
(11 OCLOCK)
BABS PICKED UP
11 OCLOCK
JACK INDOORS
TODAY
A WONKY DONKY
BABS
SHOPS.

July 13th

Jack has noted that his son-in-law, Paul, had rung, and that he went out to lunch. I feel like it could have given him a sense of satisfaction to be able to say that the housework was done, as he's noted it down on the next page.

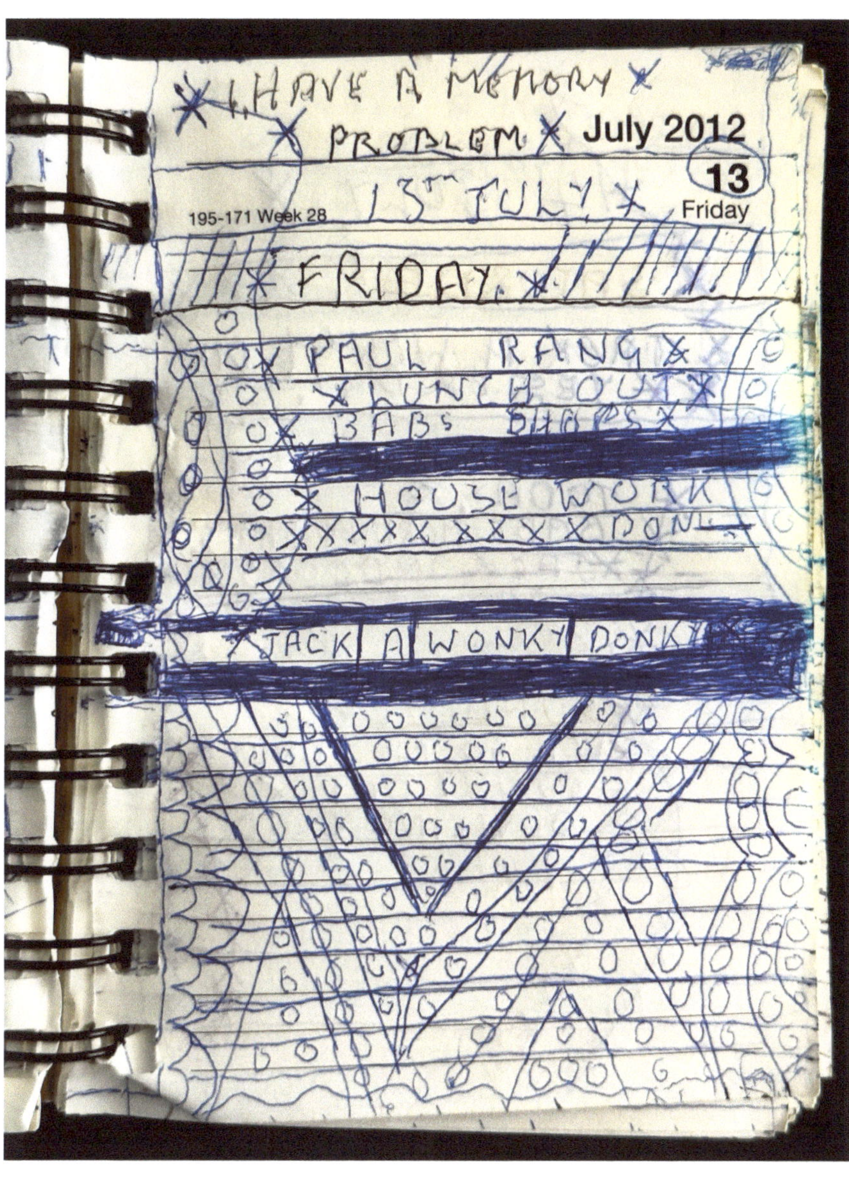
✻ I HAVE A MEMORY ✻
PROBLEM ✻ July 2012
195-171 Week 28   13TH JULY ✻   13 Friday
✻ FRIDAY. ✻
✻ PAUL RANG ✻
✻ LUNCH OUT ✻
✻ BABS SHOPS ✻
✻ HOUSE WORK
XXXXX XXX X DONE
JACK A WONKY DONKY

July 16th

Babs's hairdresser is coming to the house to do her hair today. Jack still manages a little smiley face even though he prefers it when it is just himself and Babs at home.

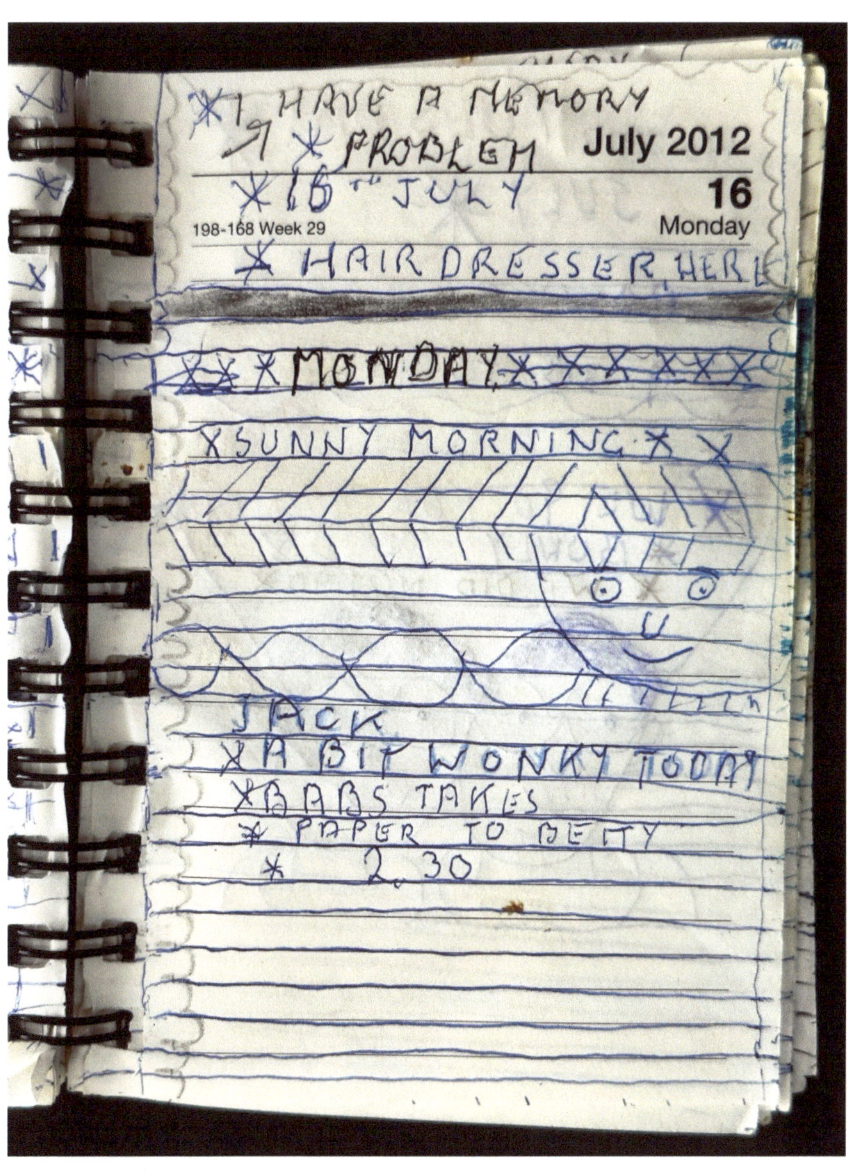
* I HAVE A MEMORY
* PROBLEM
July 2012
* 16TH JULY
16
Monday
198-168 Week 29
* HAIRDRESSER HERE
* * * MONDAY * * * * * *
* SUNNY MORNING * *
JACK
* A BIT WONKY TODAY
* BABS TAKES
* PAPER TO BETTY
* 2.30

July 26th

It feels like this wasn't a great day for Jack. As I mentioned on the last page you read, I don't think he was keen on days when 'others' came to the house. But by this stage, Babs needed help with the housework, so it was inevitable that Jack was going to have to put up with others more of the time than he would have liked.

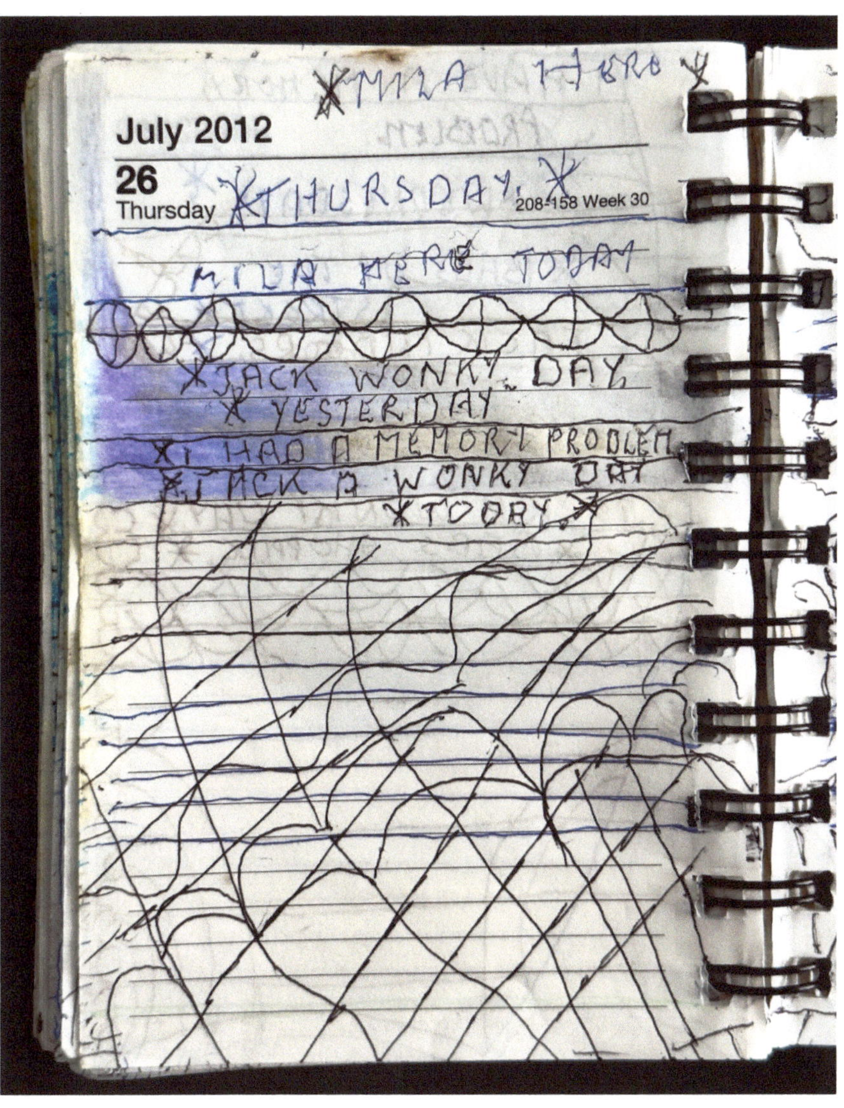

MILA HERE PROBLEM
July 2012
26 Thursday THURSDAY 208-158 Week 30
MILA HERE TODAY
JACK WONKY DAY
YESTERDAY
I HAD A MEMORY PROBLEM
JACK A WONKY DAY
TODAY

July 27th

Jack has noted that Babs had a 'hearing aid' appointment.

It's interesting to note that there's an asterisk against each entry. I wonder if the asterisks help Jack to 'take control' of his day. You'll notice that he does this more often than not.

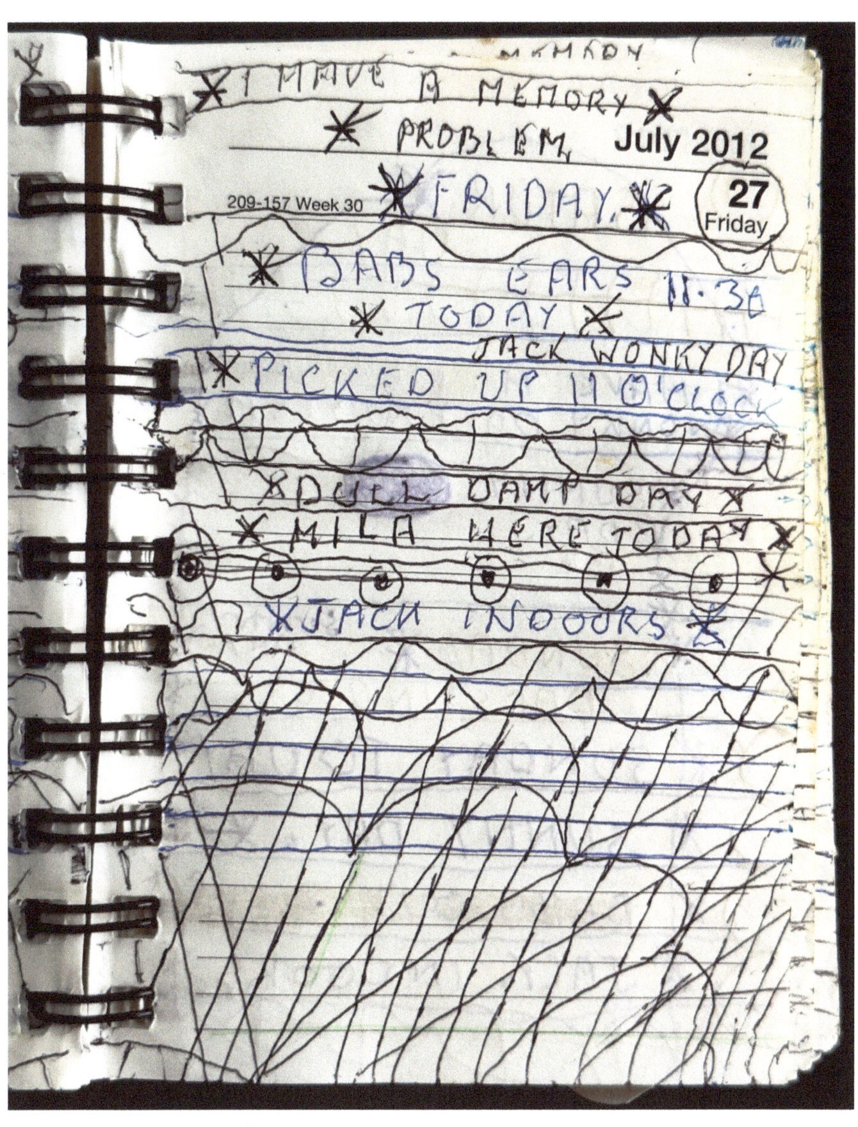
I HAVE A MEMORY
PROBLEM
July 2012
209-157 Week 30 FRIDAY
27 Friday
BABS EARS 11·30
TODAY
JACK WONKY DAY
PICKED UP 11 O'CLOCK
DULL DAMP DAY
MILA HERE TODAY
JACK INDOORS

August 6th

The entry for this day is just a face. I wonder if Jack was drawing himself here. As usual, he notes that he's having a wonky day and that he has a memory problem.

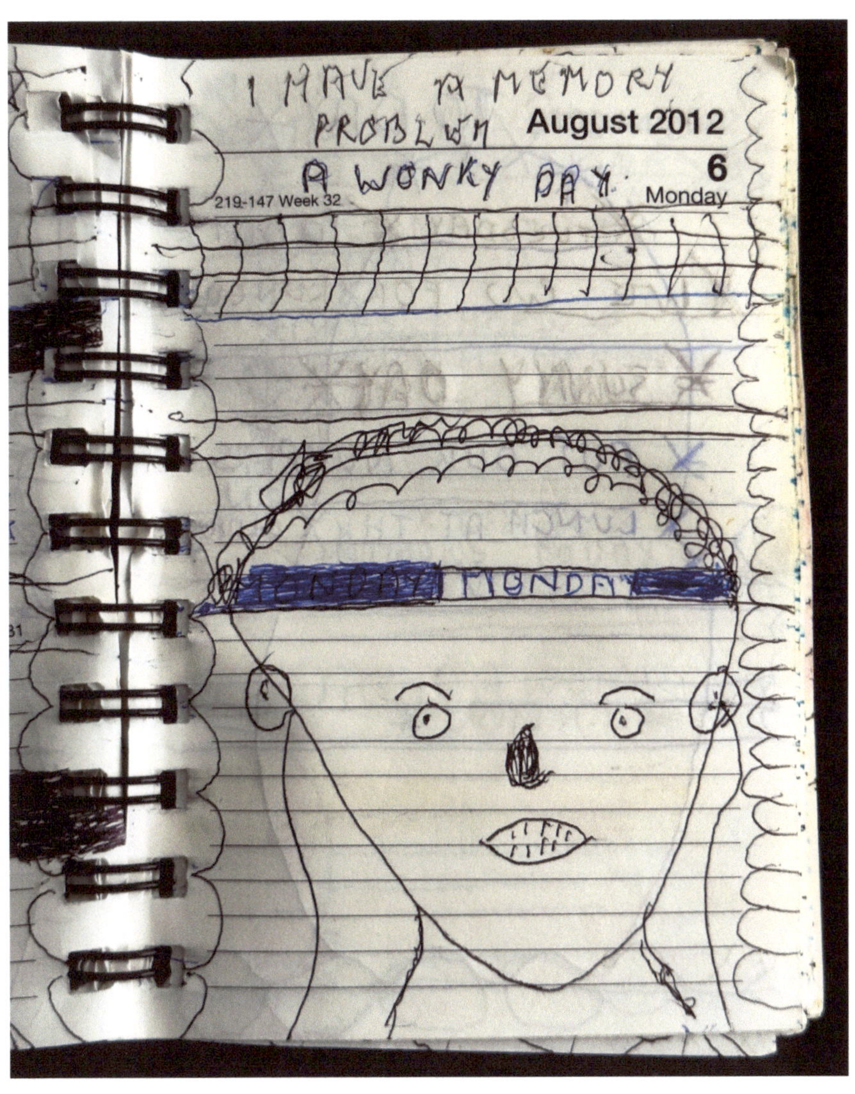
I HAVE A MEMORY
PROBLUM
A WONKY DAY
August 2012
219-147 Week 32
6
Monday
MONDAY MONDAY

August 16th

Today is Babs's birthday. Jack has noted that there's a card in the box. I suspect Babs bought the birthday card for Jack to give to her and told him where he'd be able to find it.

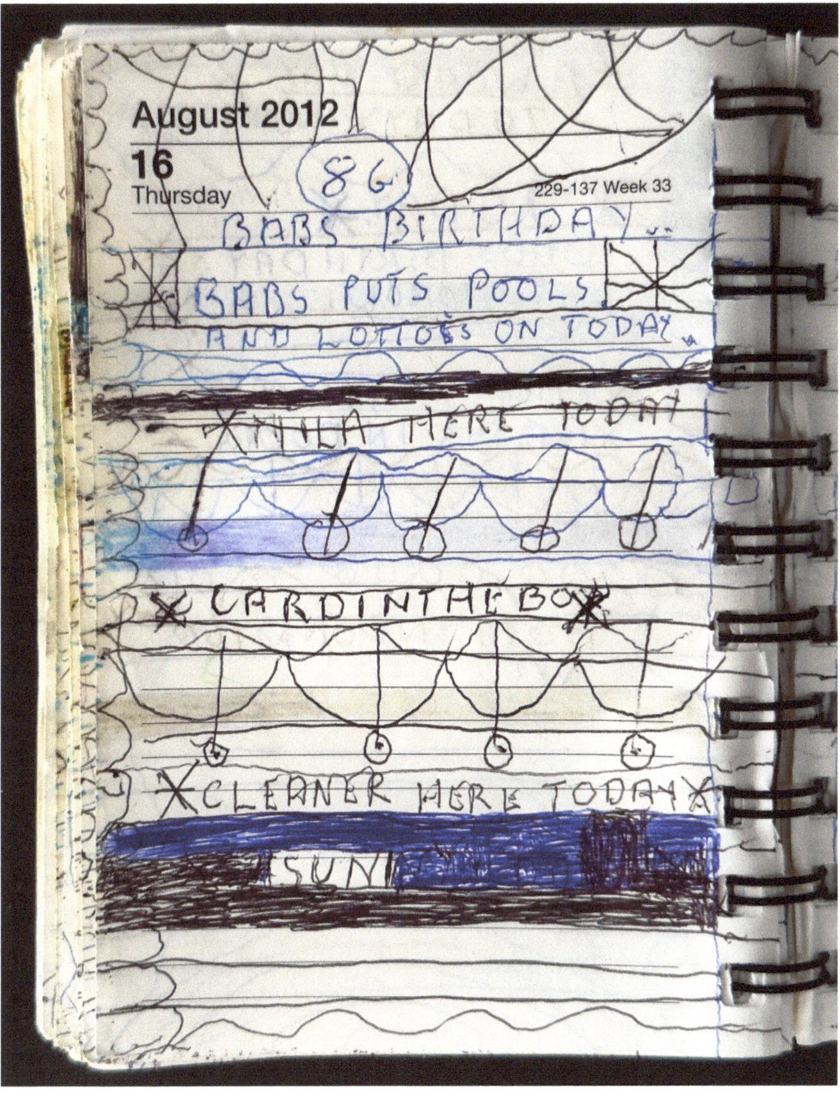
August 2012
16
Thursday
86
229-137 Week 33
BABS BIRTHDAY
BABS PUTS POOLS
AND LOTTOS ON TODAY
NULA HERE TODAY
CARDINTHEBOX
CLEANER HERE TODAY
SUN

August 21ˢᵗ

In spite of his obvious struggle with his handwriting here, it would appear that Jack enjoyed his lunch, which included crackers and cheese and a glass of veno!

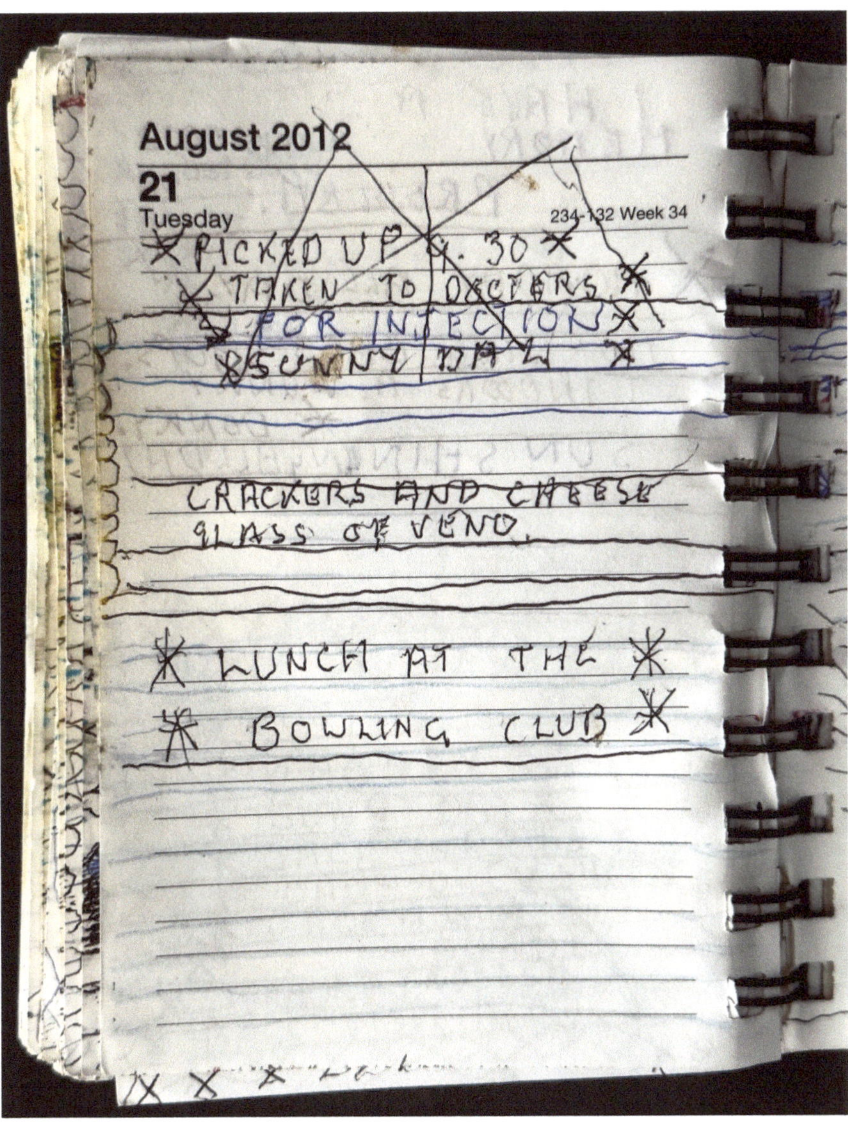

August 2012
21
Tuesday
234-132 Week 34
PICKED UP 9.30
TAKEN TO DOCTERS
FOR INJECTION
SUNNY DAY
CRACKERS AND CHEESE
GLASS OF VENO.
LUNCH AT THE
BOWLING CLUB

August 31ˢᵗ

I'm pretty certain that my sister Judy and I had a couple of glasses of veno on the day in question. Although Jack says that we went to the club, my memory of this day is that he didn't actually come out to lunch with us this time. Not that it really makes any difference in the scheme of things.

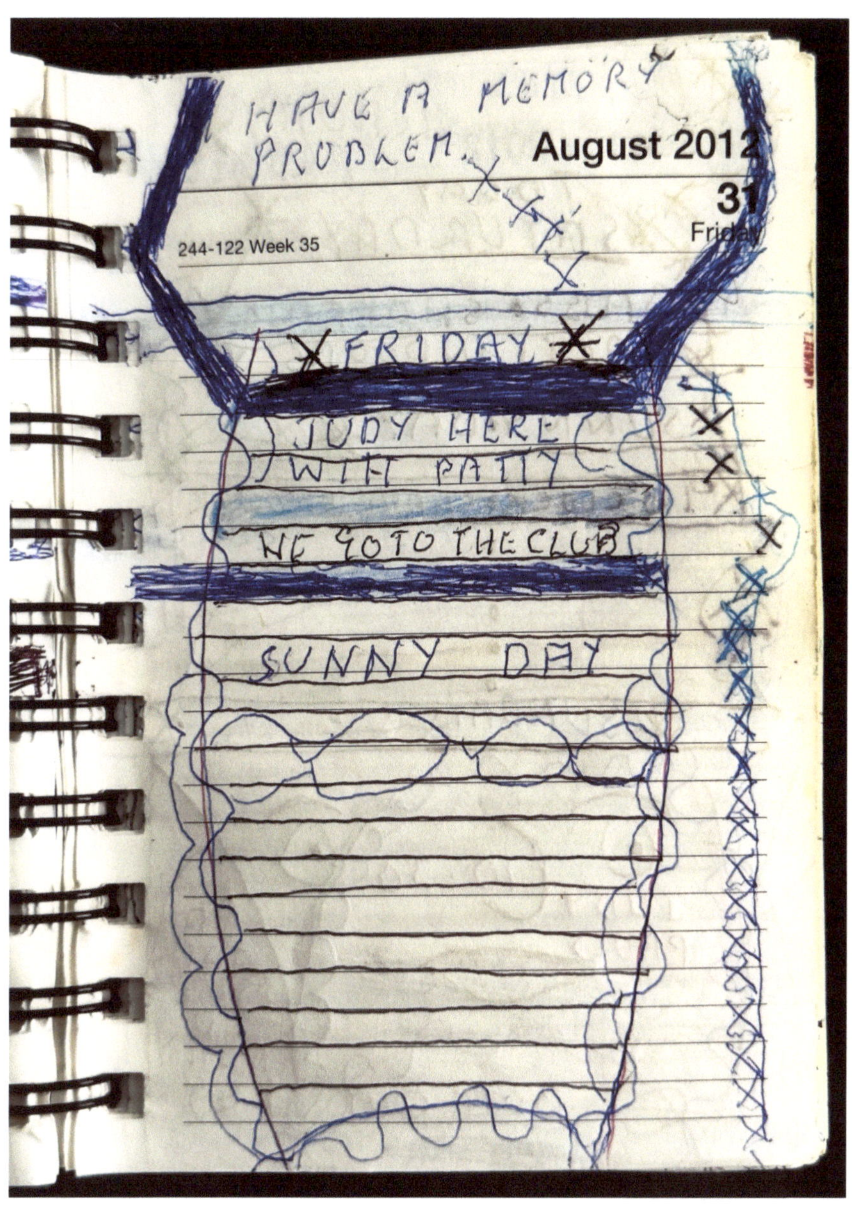
HAVE A MEMORY
PROBLEM.
August 2012
31
Friday
244-122 Week 35
FRIDAY
JUDY HERE
WITH PATTY
WE GO TO THE CLUB
SUNNY DAY

September 8th and 9th

Gone are the fun drawings and the lottery/keno numbers. In fact, Jack didn't have much to say at all. I can only wonder what was going on with him during this weekend.

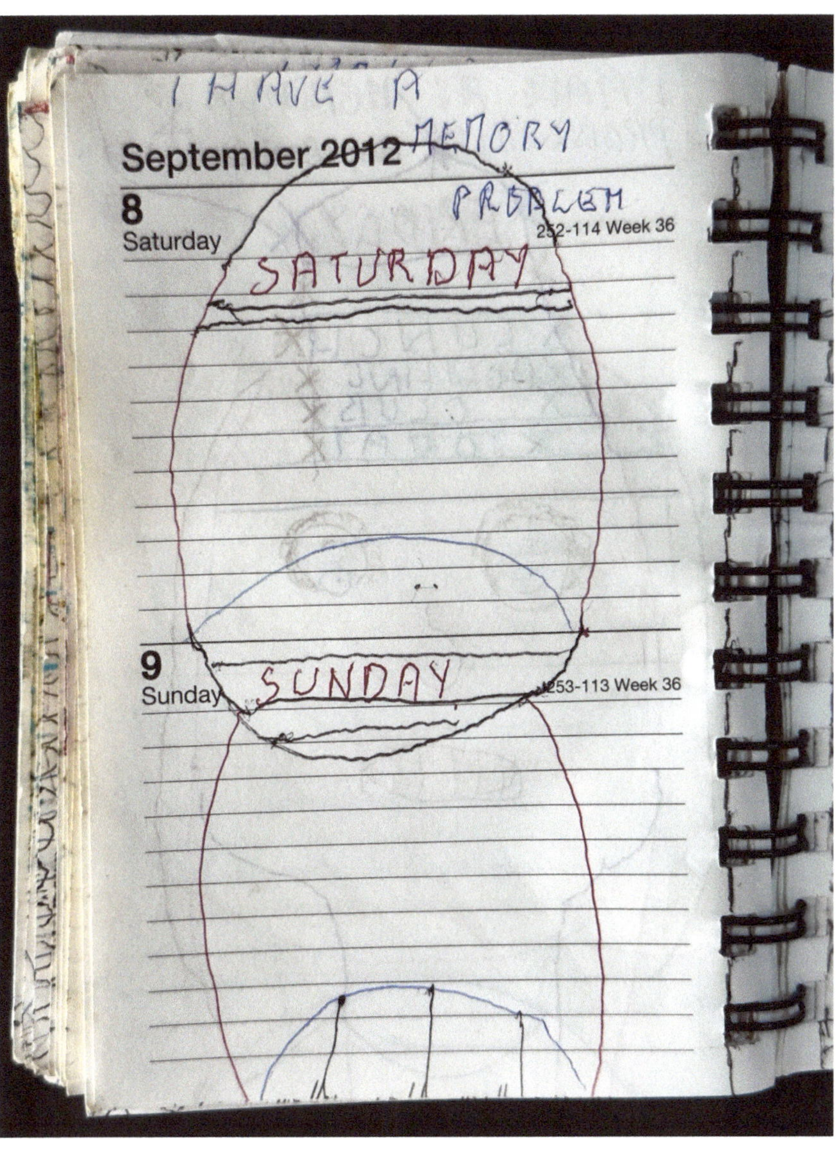

September 2012

8
Saturday

252-114 Week 36

9
Sunday

253-113 Week 36

September 24th

Jack has made quite a few entries that are easy to miss here, including the fact that it was a sunny day. You have to look hard to find those words sitting under the dark lines around the bank balance.

I smiled when I saw the proof that he really liked the 'Wonky Donkey' nickname. Today, he included a smiley face on both sides of those words.

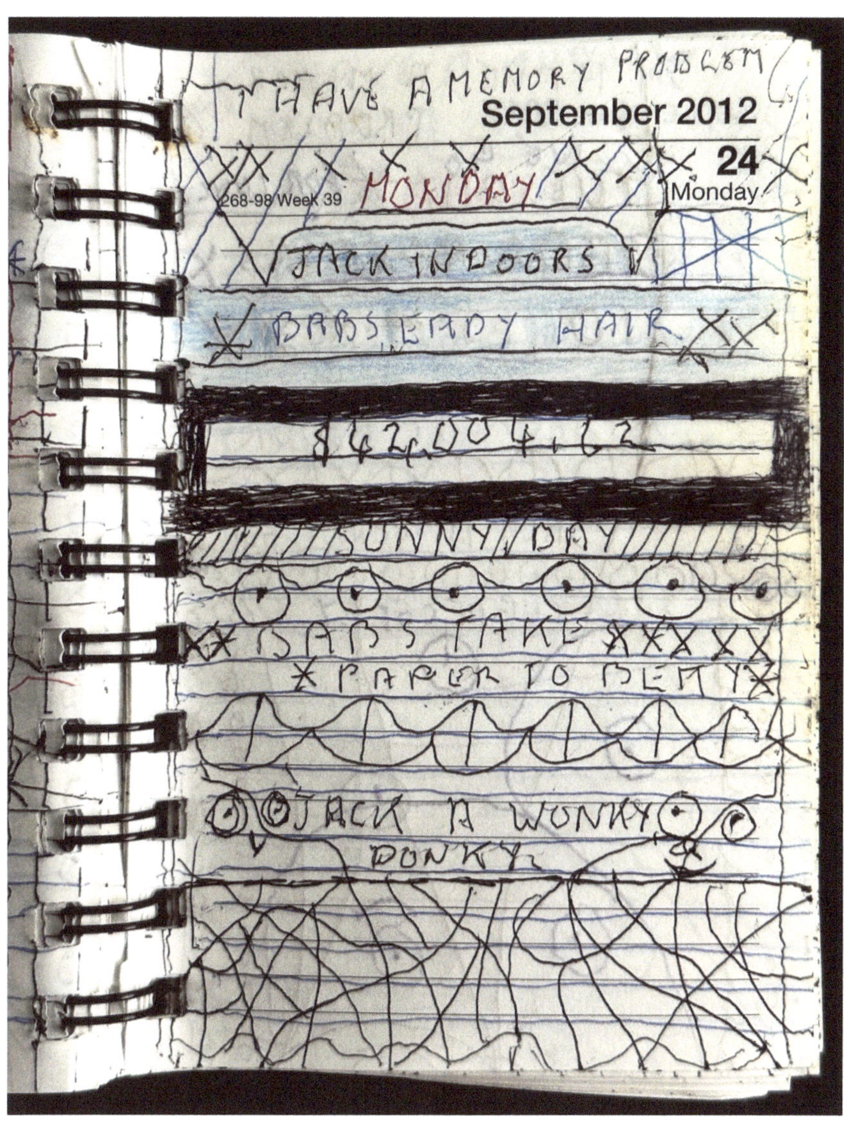
I HAVE A MEMORY PROBLEM
September 2012
268-98 Week 39   MONDAY   24 Monday
JACK INDOORS
BABS LADY HAIR
$42,004.62
SUNNY DAY
BABS TAKE PAPER TO DEMY
JACK A WONKY DONKY

October 1st

Jack continues to record their bank balance and call himself a Wonky Donkey.

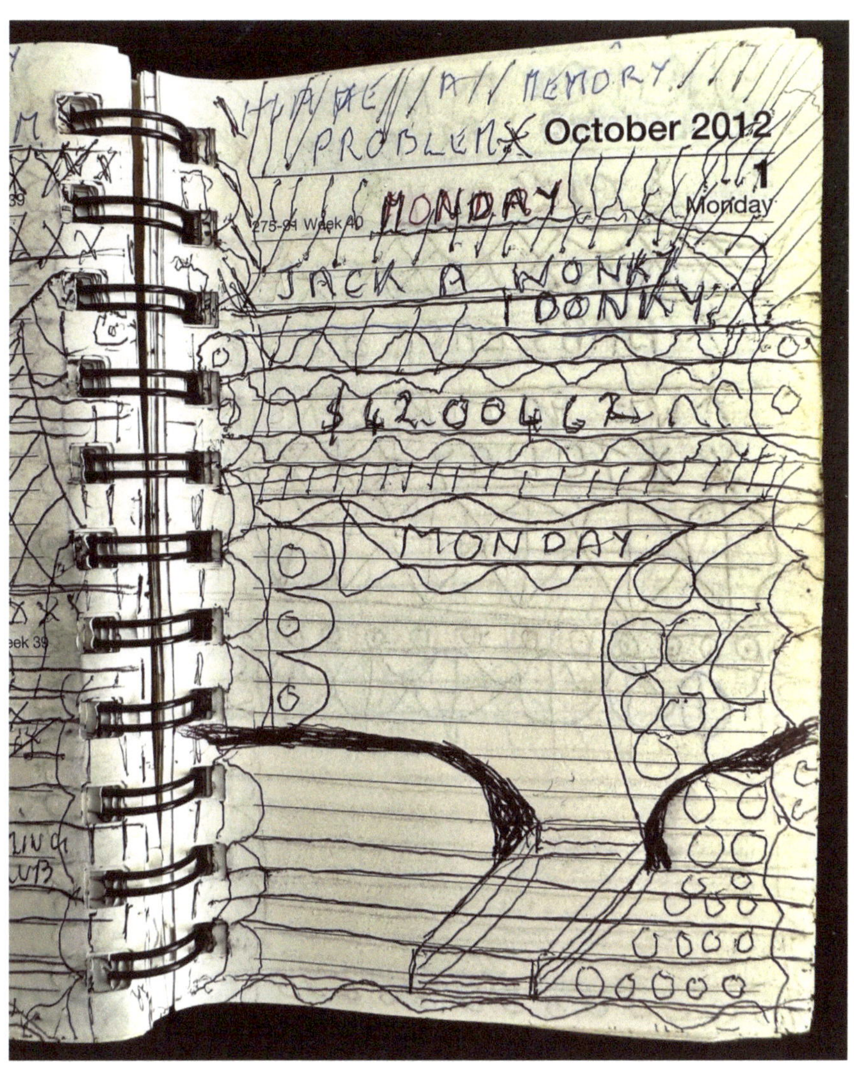
MEMORY
PROBLEM
October 2012
MONDAY
275-91 Week 40
Monday
1
JACK A WONK DONKY
$42.00 4 GR
MONDAY
Week 39

October 21st

This day turned out to be Jack's last birthday. He and Babs joined my sister Judy at the Engadine Bowling Club to celebrate his birthday with him.

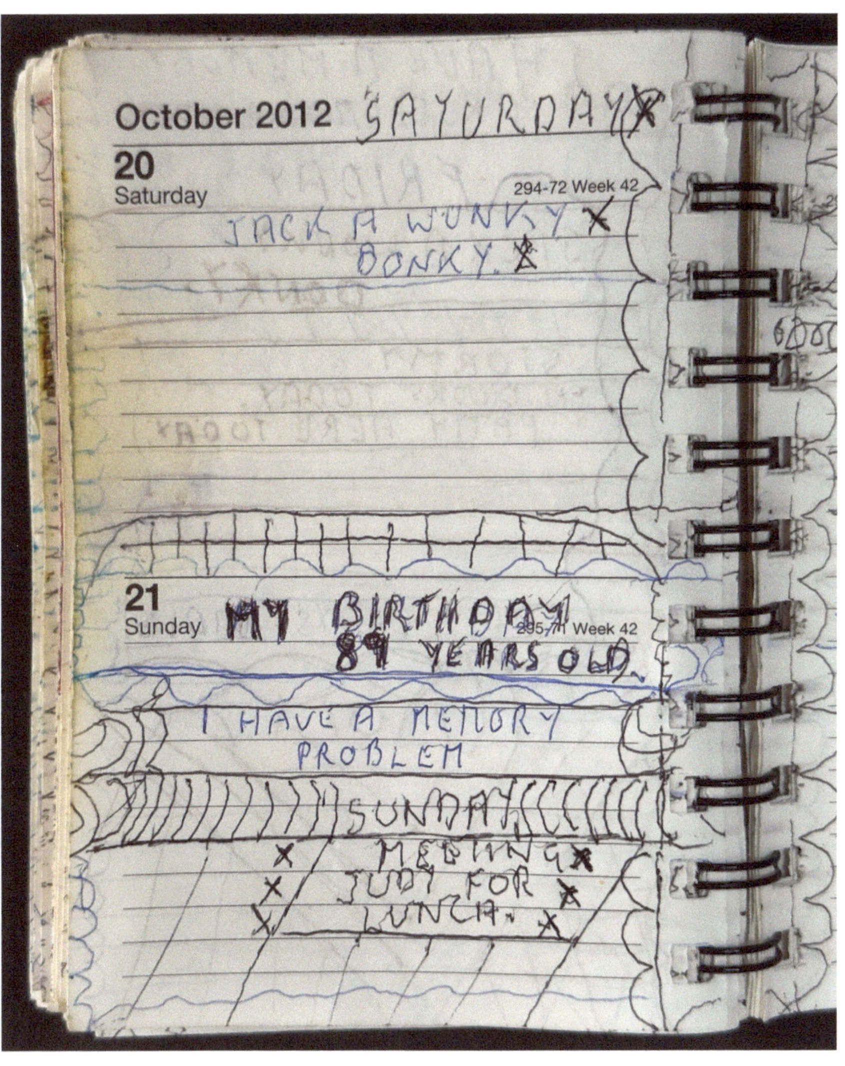
October 2012
20
Saturday
294-72 Week 42
SAYURDAY
JACK A WONKY
BONKY.
21
Sunday
295-71 Week 42
MY BIRTHDAY
89 YEARS OLD.
I HAVE A MEMORY
PROBLEM
SUNDAY
MEETING
JUDY FOR
LUNCH.

October 29th

I feel like this must have been a difficult day for Jack. He's struggling to put words on the page, but perhaps the movement of the pen on the page gave him some comfort.

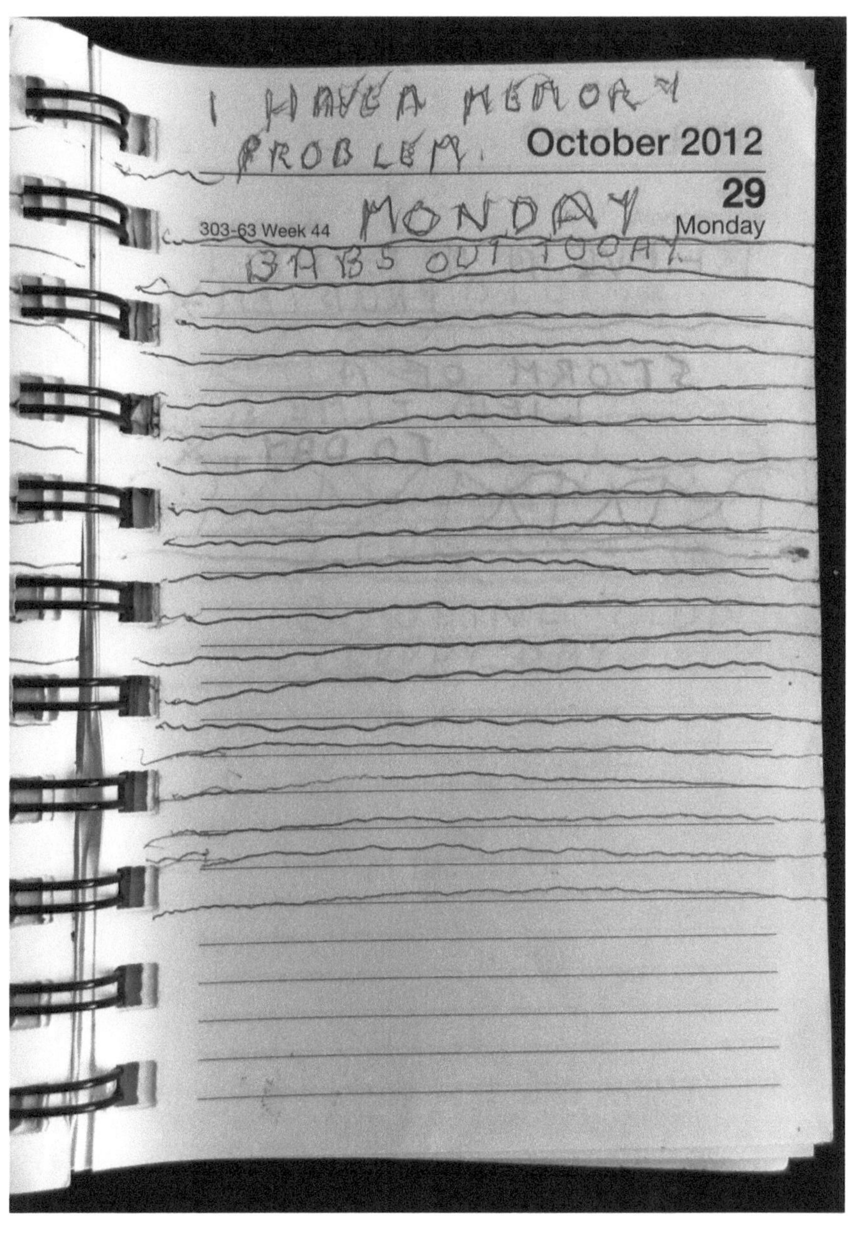
I HAVE A MEMORY
PROBLEM
October 2012
303-63 Week 44
MONDAY
29
Monday
BABS OUT TODAY

November 16th

We all love crackers and cheese!

This was a better day for Jack. Meanwhile, his writing is becoming more laboured. That said, he was still able to record the fact that his daughters were visiting that day, and that there would be crackers and cheese involved.

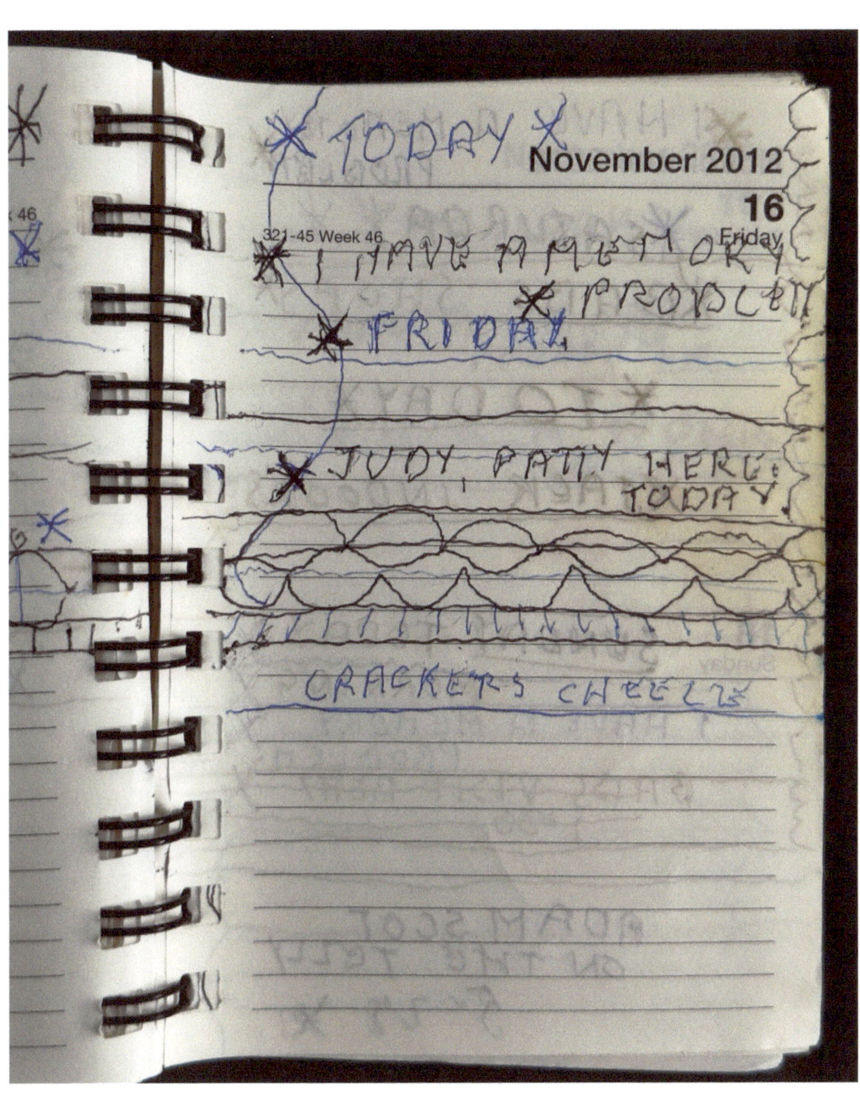
TODAY
November 2012
16
Friday
321-45 Week 46
I HAVE A MEMORY PROBLEM
FRIDAY
JUDY, PATTY HERE TODAY
CRACKERS CHEEZ

December 25th

This was Jack's last Christmas. He was still happily living at home with his beloved Babs at this stage. In those days, family members would be popping in for most of the day, wishing them a happy Christmas.

Jack remained at home until early 2013 when he became unwell and was taken to hospital, and subsequently to a care home where he passed away on Anzac Day, April 25th, 2013.

What you'll find on the next couple of pages are some of the things I wish I'd known when Jack was first diagnosed with dementia. I hope you find it helpful in some way.

I HAVE A MEMORY PROBLEM.
December 2012
25
Tuesday
460-06 Week 52
XMRSDAY X
XTUESDAY X
XTODAY X

Chapter 8

Things To Consider

Caring for someone with dementia is a profoundly challenging and rewarding journey, marked by constant learning and adaptation. Dementia is a broad term for conditions characterised by a decline in memory, reasoning, and other thinking skills. It's fair to say that, to some degree or other, it negatively impacts the daily lives of those it touches. As a caregiver, a concerned friend, a family member, or someone with dementia, I feel like understanding the nuances of the condition helps when it comes to providing compassionate support and maintaining your own well-being.

Here are some of the insights I've picked up along the way that I'm hoping will help anyone who has dementia, or is being touched by it in some way or other.

Understanding the Condition: While Alzheimer's disease is the most common form, others like vascular dementia, Lewy body dementia, and frontotemporal dementia have their own unique symptoms. Organisations like the Alzheimer's Association provide valuable information for anyone who needs it.

Recognising Symptoms: As with most conditions, early detection can be very beneficial. Things to be on the lookout for are memory loss, difficulty performing complex tasks, language difficulties, disorientation, and changes in mood or behaviour.

Progression Awareness: Dementia is typically progressive, so understanding that changes will occur can help caregivers prepare for future needs and make necessary adjustments in arrangements around quality of life and safety.

Modifying Communication: Using simple words and sentences, as well as speaking slowly and clearly, is the way to go. Don't forget that body language, facial expressions, and tone of voice play a big role in communication as well as the words we speak. Positive verbal and non-verbal communication can provide comfort and reduce anxiety in the event of stress building up. Don't forget the power of really paying attention and being present. This is important because in a lot of cases, it takes people with dementia longer to process information and respond than it takes other folk.

Triggers to be aware of: Changes in the environment, health issues, or even certain times of the day can trigger distress. Being aware of these kinds of triggers and mitigating them wherever possible can make a big difference to the quality of life for both the carer and the person being cared for.

Creating a Routine: A consistent daily routine can be particularly helpful because it creates a sense of stability and security for people with dementia. Basically, anything that can reduce confusion and agitation has to be a good thing.

Providing Engaging Activities: Activities that match the individual's abilities and interests can enhance their quality of life. These might include music, art, puzzles, or walking in nature.

Creating a Safe and Nurturing Environment: Modifying the living environment to minimise risks by doing things like installing grab bars, removing trip hazards, and using safety devices as necessary, is important where issues with stability and mobility become apparent. It goes without saying that ensuring physical needs are met with a healthy diet, hydration, a comfortable living space, and regular medical check-ups is also important.

Self-Care for the Caregiver: Caregiving can be emotionally and physically draining. It is critical to prioritise your own health and well-being through regular breaks, exercising, and social activities, as well as seeking help whenever you need it if you are the one doing the caring. Joining caregiver support groups, either in-person or online, can be a really effective way to gain emotional support and practical advice. And don't hesitate to seek help from healthcare professionals, including doctors, nurses, and social workers, if you ever feel like you're a bit lost or overwhelmed. These professionals can offer guidance, support services, and possibly even respite options for you to consider.

Empathy and Reassurance: People with dementia often feel vulnerable. Providing emotional support, reassurance, and comfort is crucial to helping them feel safe and valued. It's important to celebrate the person and focus on what they can do with their remaining strengths, rather than fixating on what they've lost. There's a whole lot of benefit in celebrating small successes and cherishing moments of connection.

Legal and Financial Planning: It's well worth discussing and documenting any legal, financial, and end-of-life wishes early in the diagnosis. It's also worth exploring resources that can help manage the financial burden of care, such as government programs, insurance benefits, and community resources.

Caring for someone with dementia relies on compassion, patience, and resilience. It's a journey filled with challenges, but also moments of profound connection and love. Arming yourself with knowledge and support, and never losing sight of the importance of your own well-being, will set you up to fare better than staying in a place of denial ever could.

Chapter 9

Conclusion

I can't be sure of Dad's intentions when he started keeping a diary. I think it was his way of keeping track of what was going on and having a sense of control. What I do know is that he's left an important legacy in the form of his diaries that I've taken parts of to share with you here.

I'm no expert in dementia that's for sure, but I'm hoping that in some small way, I might have been able to give someone with a dementia diagnosis and/or the people who love them, a sense of what the dementia journey could look like through the recordings of the wonderful man I am proud to call my father.

As I mentioned earlier, Jack passed away on Anzac Day, April 25th, 2013.

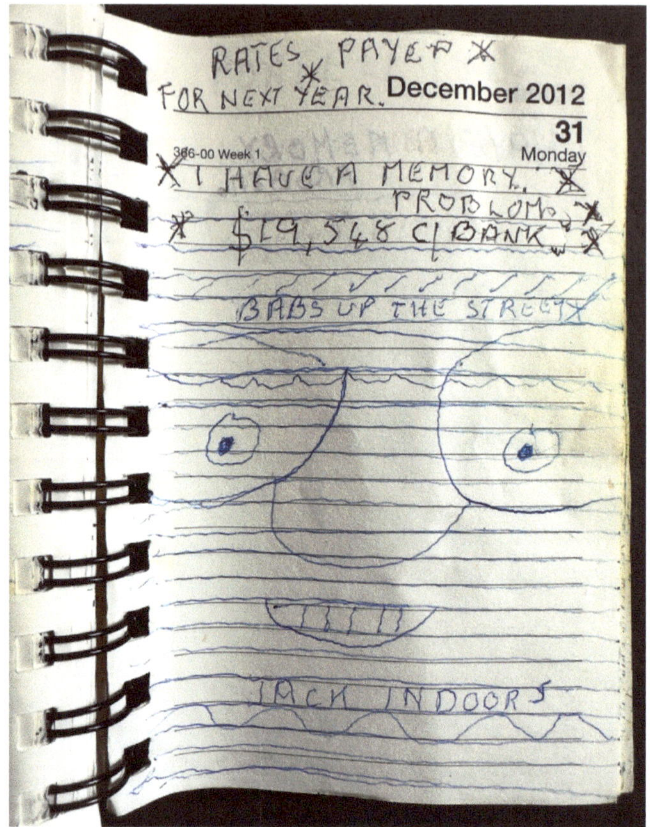

This is Jack's last diary entry. He's still recording their bank balance, and notes that the rates have been paid for the next year. I can't help but notice that this entry has a notably happy feel to it.

What you'll find on the following pages are some images that will give you a sense of the man Jack was before he was diagnosed with dementia.

Chapter 10

Appendix

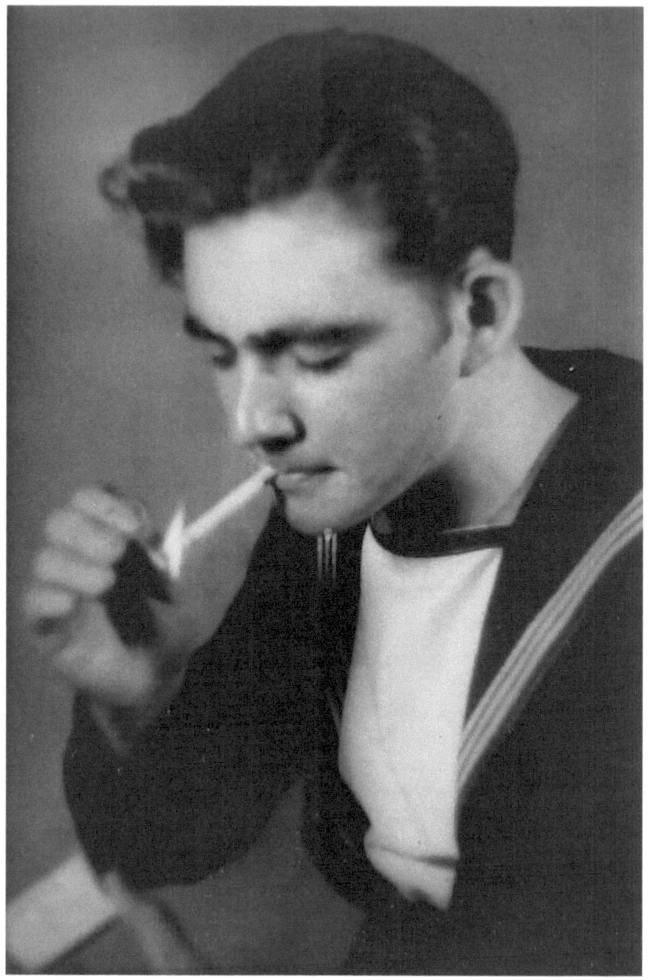

Jack joined the Royal Navy at the beginning of World War 2 until the war ended in 1939.

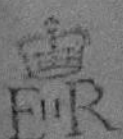

Back in 1978, Jack received this invitation to a garden party at Buckingham Palace. I guess it was in recognition of the services he provided through the role he held as a union organiser. Anything to do with royalty was an unusual thing for Jack the rebel to be involved in.

It was a pity his surname was misspelt with the 'e' that sits between the 'd' and the 's' missing, but he was used to that because it often happened. Apparently, it was an enjoyable day.

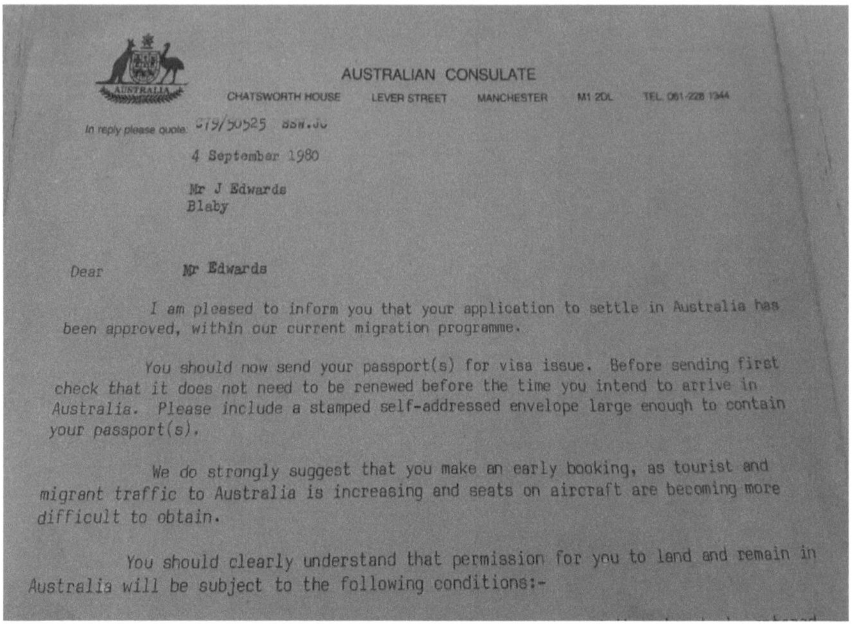

This is the long-awaited letter giving Jack and Babs permission to settle in Australia, dated 4 September 1980.

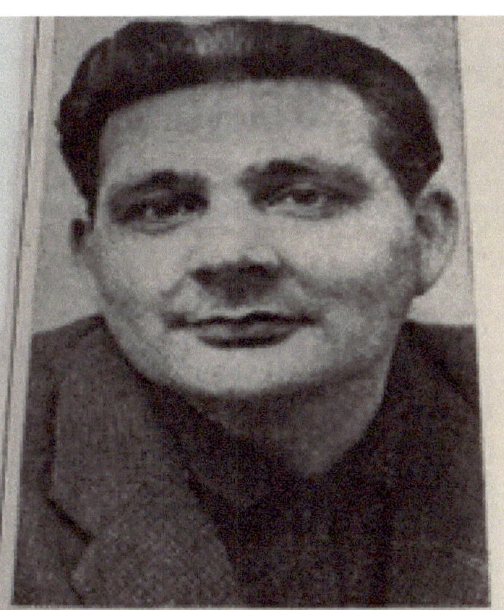

NEW ORGANISER FOR BUILDING TRADES UNION

THE new Leicester District Organiser for the Amalgamated Union of Building Trades' Workers is Mr. Jack Irving Edwardes.

Aged 40, Mr. Edwardes has been a building trade worker. He came to the Building Trade Workers from the Bricklayers' and Steelworkers' Union, in Northamptonshire, where he was an official.

A Northamptonshire man, he is married with two daughters.

Mr. Edwardes, who replaces Mr. J. H. H. Walker, now labour officer for a building firm, says he hopes to strengthen the organisation of the union in the district.

This short article dates back to 1964 when Jack was appointed to the role of Leicester District Organiser for the Amalgamated Union of Building Trades Workers. This speaks to his leadership qualities and commitment to defending the rights of workers.

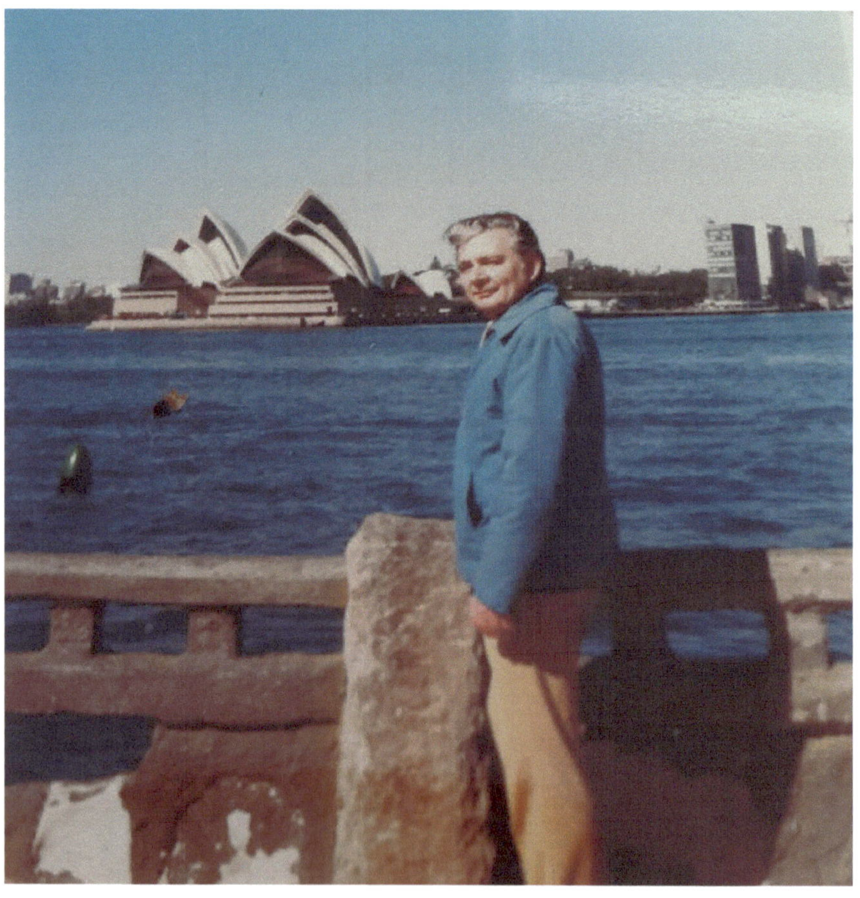

Jack loved living in Australia. He and Babs became Australian citizens on January 26th, 1985. Here he is on a beautiful sunny day with the Sydney Opera House in the background. Jack and Babs could finally be close to their daughters, sons-in-law and, later, their grandchildren.

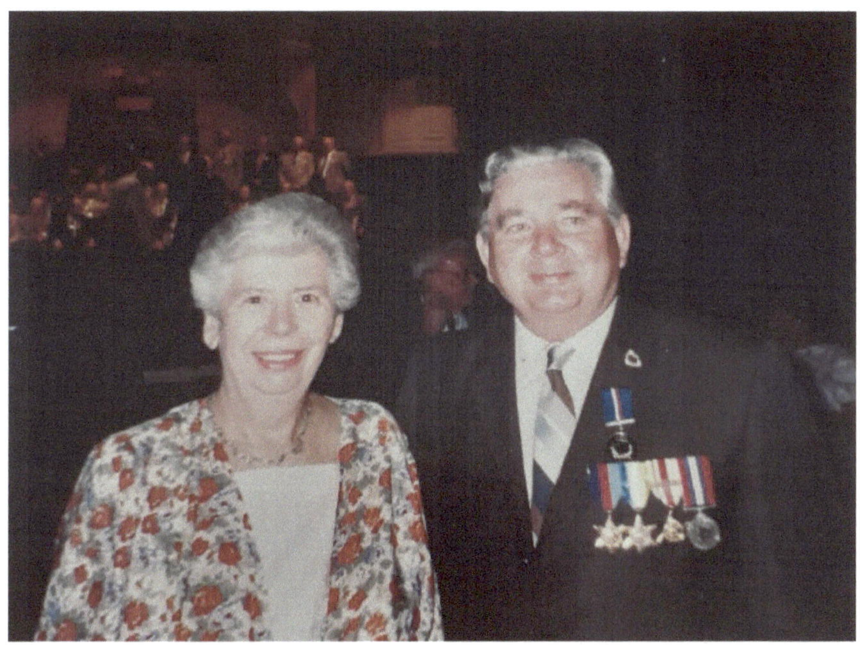

On 22/4/1993, Jack received the Malta George Cross Fiftieth Anniversary Medal at Sydney Town Hall. He was so proud, as was Babs, who was standing by his side.

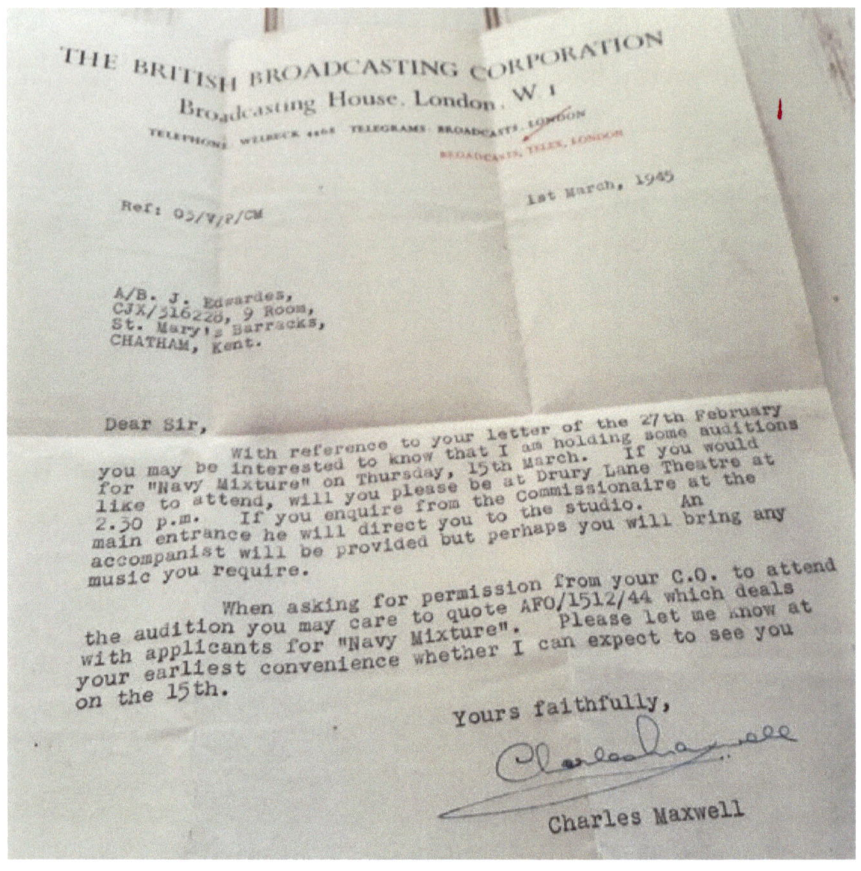

THE BRITISH BROADCASTING CORPORATION

Broadcasting House, London, W 1

TELEPHONE: WELBECK 4468   TELEGRAMS: BROADCASTS, LONDON

BROADCASTS, TELEX, LONDON

1st March, 1945

Ref: 03/V/P/CM

A/B. J. Edwardes,
CJX/516226, 9 Room,
St. Mary's Barracks,
CHATHAM, Kent.

Dear Sir,

        With reference to your letter of the 27th February
you may be interested to know that I am holding some auditions
for "Navy Mixture" on Thursday, 15th March.   If you would
like to attend, will you please be at Drury Lane Theatre at
2.30 p.m.   If you enquire from the Commissionaire at the
main entrance he will direct you to the studio.   An
accompanist will be provided but perhaps you will bring any
music you require.

        When asking for permission from your C.O. to attend
the audition you may care to quote AFO/1512/44 which deals
with applicants for "Navy Mixture".   Please let me know at
your earliest convenience whether I can expect to see you
on the 15th.

                        Yours faithfully,

                        Charles Maxwell

I found this letter among Jack's paperwork. I'd love to know more. It's a letter from the BBC (British Broadcasting Corporation) regarding auditions for their program, 'Navy Mixtures.' Jack was 23 years old at this time. To become an entertainer like his parents was most probably his ambition at this time.

About The Author

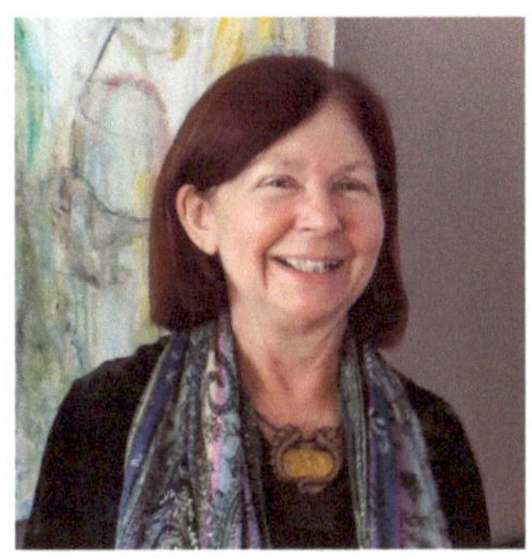

Pat lives in Scarborough on the south coast of New South Wales.

Prior to devoting her time to writing, Pat dedicated her energy to working in children's services for over 20 years. This included Early Childhood Education, Out of School Hours Care, and as the Kids' Deck Coordinator at the National Maritime Museum, as well as spending time as a TAFE teacher.

In addition to pulling "Still a Bit Wonky" together, Pat is a writer of poetry, short stories, flash fiction and children's picture books.

Her poetry has been published in children's literary magazines and has won awards in the UK and Australia.